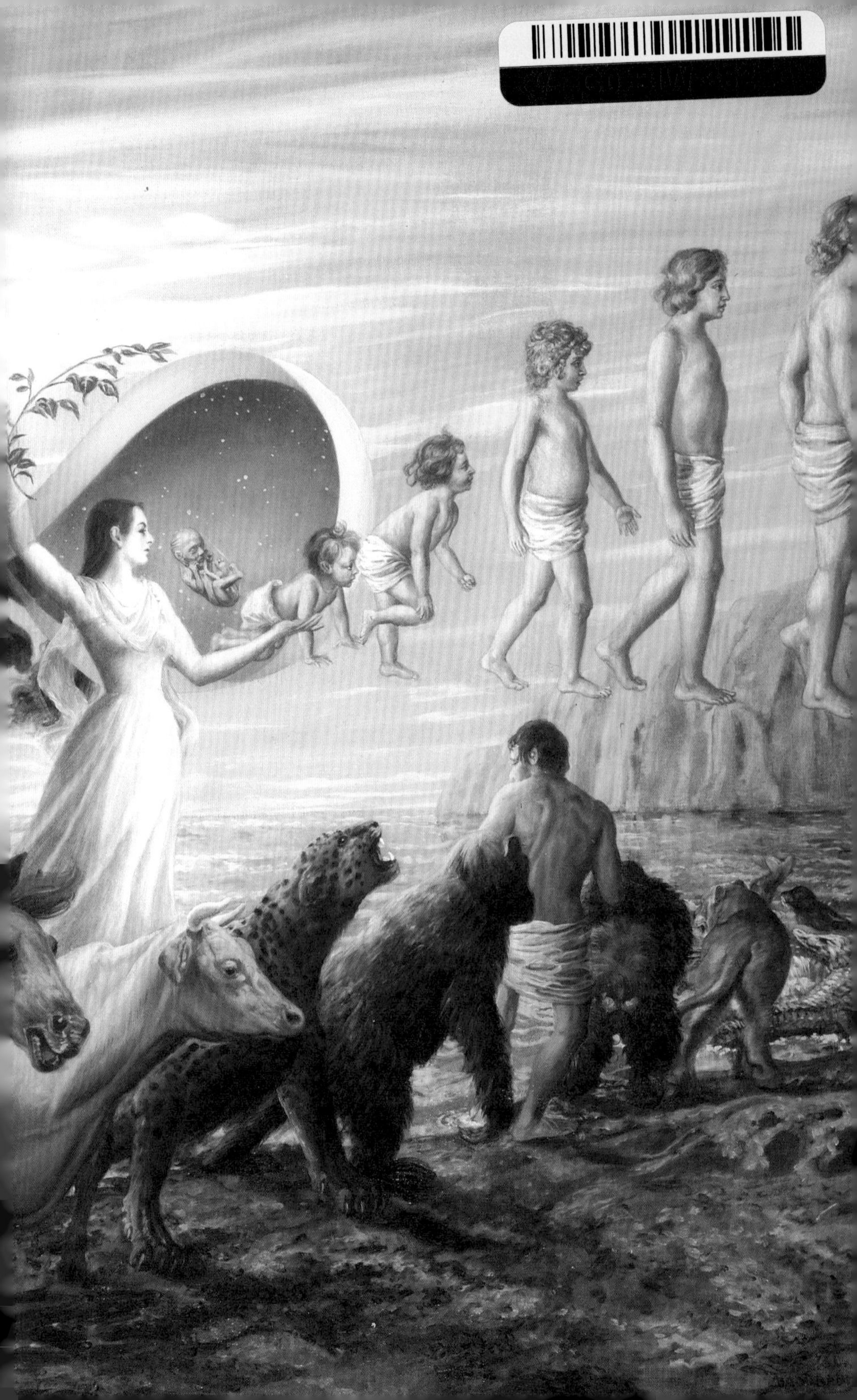

THE YOGA
OF DIVINE LOVE. . .

A world-renowned *yoga* master cuts through the commercialism that now clouds the real meaning of *yoga.*

His Divine Grace A.C. Bhaktivedanta Swami Prabhupāda explains that beyond the postures and exercises, the ancient teachings of *yoga* aim at lasting, loving union with the Supreme.

BOOKS by
His Divine Grace
A. C. Bhaktivedanta Swami Prabhupāda

Bhagavad-gītā As It Is
Śrīmad-Bhāgavatam (18 vols.; with disciples)
Śrī Caitanya-caritāmṛta (9 vols.)
The Nectar of Devotion
Kṛṣṇa, The Supreme Personality of Godhead
Teachings of Lord Caitanya
Śrī Īśopaniṣad
The Nectar of Instruction
Easy Journey to Other Planets
Kṛṣṇa Consciousness: The Topmost Yoga System
Perfect Questions, Perfect Answers
Teachings of Lord Kapila, the Son of Devahūti
Transcendental Teachings of Prahlāda Mahārāja
Dialectic Spiritualism–A Vedic View of Western Philosophy
Teachings of Queen Kuntī
Kṛṣṇa, the Reservoir of Pleasure
The Science of Self-Realization
The Path of Perfection
Search for Liberation
Life Comes from Life
The Perfection of Yoga
Beyond Birth and Death
On the Way to Kṛṣṇa
Rāja-vidyā: The King of Knowledge
Elevation to Kṛṣṇa Consciousness
Kṛṣṇa Consciousness: The Matchless Gift
The Nārada-bhakti-sūtra (with disciples)
The Mukunda-mālā-stotra (with disciples)
A Second Chance
The Journey of Self-Discovery
The Laws of Nature
Wisdom Through Renunciation
Geetār-gan (Bengali)
Vairāgya-vidyā (Bengali)
Buddhi-yoga (Bengali)
Bhakti-ratna-boli (Bengali)
Back to Godhead magazine (founder)

THE PATH OF YOGA

His Divine Grace
A. C. BHAKTIVEDANTA
SWAMI PRABHUPĀDA
FOUNDER-ĀCĀRYA OF THE INTERNATIONAL SOCIETY FOR KRISHNA CONSCIOUSNESS

THE BHAKTIVEDANTA BOOK TRUST
Los Angeles • Stockholm • Sydney • Hong Kong • Mumbai

Readers interested in the subject matter of this book are invited by the International Society for Krishna Consciousness to visit any ISKCON center worldwide (see address list in the back of this book) or to correspond with the secretary.

International Society for Krishna Consciousness
3764 Watseka Avenue
Los Angeles, CA 90034
USA

Telephone: 1-800-927-4152
Internet: http://www.harekrishna.com/ara/
E-mail: letters@iskcon.com

First published as two books: *The Perfection of Yoga*, ©1971 by The Bhaktivedanta Book Trust, and *The Path of Perfection*, ©1979 by The Bhaktivedanta Book Trust.

Second Printing 1996

Printed in Portugal

Contents

Introduction

When we see a book with a title like *The Path Yoga*, we may react with a bit of skepticism: "Oh, another book claiming to give all the answers. One more do-it-yourself enlightenment scheme." And certainly it seems that such skepticism is justified nowadays. Our natural desire for ultimate meaning, happiness, enlightenment, liberation, and salvation has become the most exploited commodity of the twentieth century, creating what one contemporary theologian termed a disastrous "seduction of the spirit." This seduction is indeed the most tragic kind of exploitation. And the unfortunate consequence of this exploitation is a kind of deadening cynicism that discourages our search for self-fulfillment and the means to attain it.

The thoughtful contemporary reader, weary of the many speculative, simplistic books that clutter the bookstore shelves and offer instant formulas for psychological or spiritual salvation, will find *The Path of Yoga* a welcome relief. Herein one will find a clear, intriguing explanation of the philosophy and practice of mankind's oldest system of spiritual development—*yoga.*

Now, the word *yoga* may conjure up an image of some skinny fakir contorted like a human pretzel, or perhaps a room full aging New Agers struggling to stand on their heads in hope of improving their health and losing weight. This is not what we mean by *yoga.* Here we are referring to an ancient philosophy and meditational system that has been practiced by millions throughout the ages. What has in modern times been reduced to a commercially exploited technique of physical agility and pseudo meditation was once a comprehensive and easily applied form of self-realization.

The Path of Yoga combines two books previously published separately—*The Path of Perfection* and *The Perfection of Yoga.* These books are based on a historic series of talks given in the late 1960's by His Divine Grace A. C. Bhaktivedanta Swami Prabhupāda (1896–1977) on India's greatest spiritual classic, the *Bhagavad-gītā.* In these absorbing talks Śrīla Prabhupāda deeply explores the philosophy of *yoga* as explained in the Sixth and Eighth Chapters of the *Gītā,* showing clearly how these timeless teachings apply to the modern world. Śrīla Prabhupāda's talks probe questions concerning the nature of consciousness, techniques of meditation, *karma,* death, reincarnation, and even spiritual ecstasy.

The *Bhagavad-gītā,* described by one contemporary psychologist as "a remarkable psychotherapeutic session," appears to us in the form of an extraordinary dialog between Lord Kṛṣṇa, the Supreme Personality of Godhead, and His warrior disciple Arjuna. Confused about his identity and purpose, Arjuna turns to Kṛṣṇa, who reveals "the path of perfection" to His able student. The essence of Lord Kṛṣṇa's teachings is that one must become a *yogī,* that is, one whose life is centered on the practice of *yoga.* And what is *yoga*? The Sanskrit word *yoga* literally means "union," and it refers to the union, in love, between the individual consciousness and the Supreme Consciousness, the self and the Superself, the soul and God. The process of *yoga* Lord Kṛṣṇa describes in the *Bhagavad-gītā* is indeed the path of perfection, for it aims toward this most exalted human attainment.

In the *Bhagavad-gītā* we learn of four basic varieties of *yoga. Karma-yoga* is the process whereby one performs his work for God, without any desire for personal gain. *Jñāna-yoga* is the process of elevating oneself to spiritual consciousness by cultivating philosophical knowledge. The *aṣṭāṅga-yoga* system, of which the modern "*haṭha-yoga*" is a watered-down version, is a mechanical, meditative practice meant to control the mind and senses and focus one's concentration on the Supreme. These three *yoga* systems culminate in *bhakti-yoga,* the *yoga* of selfless, ecstatic devotional love of God, Kṛṣṇa. Lord Kṛṣṇa Himself states in the last verse of Chapter Six, "Of all *yogīs,* the one with great faith who always abides in Me, thinks of Me within himself, and renders transcendental loving service to Me—he is the most intimately united with Me in *yoga* and is the highest of all."

In *The Path of Yoga* Śrīla Prabhupāda offers a brilliant summary of the methods of *bhakti-yoga,* revealing the universal applicability of this simple but all-inclusive form of *yoga.* He shows how even those who are entangled in the complexity and chaos of modern materialistic life can begin an uncomplicated practice that purifies the mind and puts one in touch with the Supreme Consciousness.

Making the process of *bhakti-yoga* accessible to everyone in the modern world was Śrīla Prabhupāda's greatest contribution to our age. Śrīla Prabhupāda was an acknowledged master scholar of India's ancient spiritual culture and of its linguistic foundation, the Sanskrit language. But he was not a mere textual scholar or philosopher or theologian spinning out interesting philosophical or theological notions. He was a true spiritual genius who succeeded in bringing to life the essence of India's universal spiritual wisdom in a form that twentieth century men and women can easily understand and practice. This was the unique genius who inspired the late prime minister of India, Sri Lal Bahadur Shastri, to declare that the writings of Śrīla Prabhupāda "are a significant contribution to the salvation of mankind." The transforming quality of Śrīla Prabhupāda's writings was also appreciated by sociologist Elwin H. Powell, who commented on Śrīla Prabhupāda's best-selling edition of the *Bhagavad-gītā:* "This transcendental mysticism from the East is now taking root in the 'countercultures' of the West and providing for many a way out of the wilderness of a disintegrating civilization. . . . If truth is what works, there must be a kind of truth in the *Bhagavad-gītā As It Is,* since those who follow its teachings display a joyous serenity usually missing in the bleak and strident lives of contemporary people."

—*The Publishers*

PART ONE: THE PATH OF PERFECTION

1

Yoga as Action

In the Sixth and Eighth Chapters of the *Bhagavad-gītā,* Lord Śrī Kṛṣṇa, the Supreme Personality of Godhead, explains that the eightfold *yoga* system is a means to control the mind and senses. This method, however, is very difficult for people to perform, especially in the present Age of Kali, an age characterized by ignorance and chaos.

Although the eightfold *yoga* system is recommended in the Sixth Chapter of the *Bhagavad-gītā,* the Lord emphasizes that the process of *karma-yoga,* action in Kṛṣṇa consciousness, is superior. In this world everyone works to maintain his family and household, and no one is working without some self-interest, or desire for personal sense gratification, be it concentrated or extended. But to act perfectly is to act in Kṛṣṇa consciousness, and this means acting without a view to enjoying the fruits of one's labor.

It is our duty to act in Kṛṣṇa consciousness because we are constitutionally parts and parcels of the Supreme. The parts of the body work for the satisfaction of the entire body, not to satisfy the individual parts. The goal is the satisfaction of the complete whole. Similarly, the living entity should act for the satisfaction of the supreme whole, the Supreme Personality of Godhead, and not for his own personal satisfaction. One who can do this is the perfect *sannyāsī* (renunciant) and the perfect *yogī.* In the first verse of the Sixth Chapter of the *Bhagavad-gītā,* the chapter dealing with *sāṅkhya-yoga,* Bhagavān Śrī Kṛṣṇa states,

anāśritaḥ karma-phalaṁ kāryaṁ karma karoti yaḥ
sa sannyāsī ca yogī ca na niragnir na cākriyaḥ

"One who is unattached to the fruits of his work and who works as he is obligated is in the renounced order of life, and he is the true mystic, not he who lights no fire and performs no duty."

Sometimes *sannyāsīs* incorrectly think that they have become liberated from all material duties and therefore no longer have to perform *agni-hotra yajñas*, or fire sacrifices. This is a mistake. Certain *yajñas* (sacrifices) have to be performed by everyone for purification. Since *sannyāsīs* are not traditionally required to perform *yajñas*, they sometimes think that they can attain liberation by ceasing to perform the ritualistic *yajñas*, but actually, unless one comes to the platform of Kṛṣṇa consciousness, there is no question of liberation. Those *sannyāsīs* who cease to perform *yajñas* are in fact acting out of self-interest, because their goal is to become one with the impersonal Brahman. That is the ultimate goal of the impersonalists (Māyāvādīs), who have one major goal or demand: to become one with the supreme impersonal Being. The devotees have no such demands. They are simply satisfied in serving Kṛṣṇa for the satisfaction of Kṛṣṇa. They do not want anything in return. That is the characteristic of pure devotion.

It was Lord Caitanya Mahāprabhu who expressed this devotional attitude so succinctly:

na dhanaṁ na janaṁ na sundarīṁ
kavitāṁ vā jagad-īśa kāmaye
mama janmani janmanīśvare
bhavatād bhaktir ahaitukī tvayi

"O Almighty Lord, I have no desire to accumulate wealth, nor to enjoy beautiful women. Nor do I want any number of followers. I only want the causeless mercy of Your devotional service in My life, birth after birth." (*Śikṣāṣṭaka* 4) In essence, this is the *bhakti-yoga* system. There are many examples of this pure devotional attitude. Once Lord Nṛsiṁhadeva told Prahlāda Mahārāja, "My dear boy, you have suffered so much for Me. Whatever you want, ask for it." Being a pure devotee, Prahlāda Mahārāja refused to ask for anything. He said, "My dear Master, I am not carrying out mercantile business with You. I will not accept any remuneration for my service." This is the pure devotional attitude.

Yogīs and *jñānīs* are demanding to become one with the Supreme because they have such bitter experience suffering the material pangs. They want to become one with the Lord because they are suffering in separation. A pure devotee, however, does not experience this suffering. Although separate from the Lord, he fully enjoys the service of the Lord in separation. The desire to become one with the impersonal Brahman, or to merge with God, is certainly greater than any material desire, but this is not without self-interest. Similarly, the mystic *yogī* who practices the *yoga* system with half-open eyes, ceasing all material activities, desires some satisfaction for his personal self. Such *yogīs* desire material power, and that is their conception of the perfection of *yoga*. Actually, this is not the perfection of *yoga*, but a materialistic goal.

If one practices the regulative principles of *yoga*, he can attain eight kinds of perfection. He can become lighter than a cotton swab. He can become heavier than a great stone. He can immediately get whatever he likes. Sometimes he can even create a planet. Although such powers are rare nowadays, there actually exist some *yogīs* who have attained them. Viśvāmitra Yogī wanted to beget a man from a palm tree. He was thinking, "Why should a man have to live so many months within the womb of his mother? Why can't he be produced just like a fruit?" Thinking like this, Viśvāmitra Yogī produced men like coconuts. Sometimes *yogīs* are so powerful that they can perform such acts, but these are all material powers. Ultimately such *yogīs* are vanquished, because they cannot retain these material powers indefinitely.

Bhakti-yogīs, however, are not interested in such powers. The *bhakti-yogī*, acting in Kṛṣṇa consciousness, works for the satisfaction of the whole without self-interest. A Kṛṣṇa conscious person does not desire self-satisfaction. Rather, his criterion of success is the satisfaction of Kṛṣṇa; therefore he is considered the perfect *sannyāsī* and the perfect *yogī*.

A pure devotee does not even want salvation. The salvationists want to be saved from rebirth, and the voidists also want to put an end to all material life. Caitanya Mahāprabhu, however, requested only devotional service to Lord Kṛṣṇa, birth after birth; in other words, Caitanya Mahāprabhu was prepared to endure material miseries in one body after another. What, then, was Caitanya Mahāprabhu's desire? He wanted to engage in God's service, and nothing more, for that is the real perfection of *yoga*.

Whether in the spiritual sky or the material sky, the individual spirit soul is constitutionally the same. It is said that he is one ten-thousandth part of the tip of a hair. This means that our position is that of a small particle. But spirit can expand. Just as we develop a material body in the material world, we develop a spiritual body in the spiritual world. In the material world, expansion takes place in contact with matter. In the spiritual world, this expansion is spiritual.

Actually, the first lesson of the *Bhagavad-gītā* is "I am a spirit soul. I am different from the body." The spirit soul is a living force, but the material body is not. It is dull matter, and it is activated only because the spiritual force is present. In the spiritual world, everything is living force; there is no dead matter. There, the body is totally spiritual. One may compare the spirit soul with oil and the body with water. When oil is in water, there is a distinction, and that distinction always remains. In the spiritual sky, there is no question of oil being placed in water. There everything is spirit.

The impersonalists do not want to develop a spiritual body. They simply want to remain spiritual particles, and that is their idea of happiness. But we *bhakti-yogīs* (Vaiṣṇavas) want to serve Kṛṣṇa, and therefore we require hands, legs, and all the other bodily parts. So in the spiritual world we are given suitable bodies to serve Kṛṣṇa. Just as we develop a material body in our mother's womb, we can develop a spiritual body in the spiritual world.

The spiritual body is developed through the practice of Kṛṣṇa consciousness. In other words, the *bhakti-yoga* process spiritualizes the material body. If you place an iron rod within fire, the rod becomes so hot that it also becomes fiery. When the iron rod is red hot, it acquires all the qualities of fire. If you touch something with that rod, it will act as fire. Similarly, although at present our body is material, it can become spiritualized through Kṛṣṇa consciousness and act as spirit. Although copper is just a metal, as soon as it comes in contact with electricity it becomes electrified, and if you touch it you will receive an electric shock.

As soon as your body is spiritualized, material activity ceases. Material activity means acting for sense gratification. As you become spiritualized, material demands dwindle until they become nil. How is this possible? In order for an iron rod to act as fire, it must remain constantly in contact with fire. In order for the material body to become spiritualized, one must remain constantly in Kṛṣṇa consciousness. When this material body is fully engaged in spiritual activities, it becomes spiritual.

According to the Vedic system, the body of a high personality, a *sannyāsī*, is not burned but buried, because a *sannyāsī's* body is considered spiritual, having ceased to engage in material activities. If everyone in this world engages fully in Kṛṣṇa consciousness and ceases to work for sense gratification, this entire world will immediately become spiritual. Therefore it is necessary to learn how to work for the satisfaction of Kṛṣṇa. This requires a little time to understand. If something is used for Kṛṣṇa's satisfaction, it is spiritual. Since we are using microphones, typewriters, etc., in order to talk and write about Kṛṣṇa, they become spiritualized. What is the difference between *prasādam* and ordinary food? Some people may say, "What is this *prasādam*? We are eating the same food. Why do you call it *prasādam*?" It is *prasādam* because it has been offered for Kṛṣṇa's satisfaction and has thus become spiritualized.

In a higher sense, there is no matter at all. Everything is spiritual. Because Kṛṣṇa is totally spiritual and matter is one of the energies of Kṛṣṇa, matter is also spiritual. However, because the living entities are misusing this energy—that is, using it for something other than Kṛṣṇa's purposes—it becomes materialized, and so we call it matter. The purpose of the Kṛṣṇa consciousness movement is to *respiritualize* this energy. Our goal is to respiritualize the whole world—socially, politically, and in every other way. Of course, this may not be possible, but it is our ideal. At least if we individually take up this respiritualization process, our lives become perfect.

In the *Bhagavad-gītā* (9.22) Kṛṣṇa says that He provides for His devotees by giving them what they lack and preserving what they have. People are very fond of saying that God helps those who help themselves, but they do not understand that helping yourself means putting yourself under Kṛṣṇa's protection. If one thinks, "Oh, I can help myself, I can protect myself," one is thinking foolishly. Consider the analogy of the finger and the body. As long as my finger is attached to my body, it is useful, and I may spend thousands of dollars to preserve it. But if a finger is cut off, it is useless and is thrown away. Similarly, we are part and parcel of Kṛṣṇa, and helping ourselves means putting ourselves in our proper position as His parts and parcels. Otherwise, if we try to keep ourselves separate from Kṛṣṇa, how can we help ourselves? The finger can help itself only when it is situated properly on the hand and is working on behalf of the entire body. If the finger thinks, "I will separate myself from this body and help myself," that finger will be cast away and will die. As soon as we think, "I shall live independently of Kṛṣṇa," that is our spiritual death, and as soon as we engage in Kṛṣṇa's service as His part and parcel, that is our spiritual life. Therefore, helping oneself means knowing one's actual position and working accordingly. It is not possible to help oneself without knowing one's position.

Service means activity, for when we serve someone, we are acting. When we serve Kṛṣṇa, we are preaching Kṛṣṇa consciousness, or cooking, or cleansing the temple, or distributing books about Kṛṣṇa, or writing about Him, or shopping for foodstuffs to cook for Him and offer to Him. There are so many ways to serve. Serving Kṛṣṇa means acting for Him, not sitting down in one place and artificially meditating. Whatever assets we have should be utilized for Kṛṣṇa. That is the process of *bhakti-yoga,* or Kṛṣṇa consciousness. Kṛṣṇa has given us a mind, and we must utilize this mind to think of Kṛṣṇa. We have been given these hands, and we must use them to wash the temple or cook for Kṛṣṇa. We have been given these legs, and we should use them to go to the temple of Kṛṣṇa. We have been given a nose, and we should use it to smell the flowers that have been offered to Kṛṣṇa. Through the process of *bhakti-yoga,* we engage all these senses in the service of Kṛṣṇa, and in this way the senses are spiritualized.

In the *Bhagavad-gītā* Arjuna was refusing to act, and Kṛṣṇa was inspiring him to engage in activity. The entire *Bhagavad-gītā* is an inspiration to work, to engage in Kṛṣṇa consciousness, to act on Kṛṣṇa's behalf. Kṛṣṇa never tells Arjuna, "My dear friend Arjuna, don't concern yourself with this war. Just sit down and meditate upon Me." This is not the message of the *Bhagavad-gītā.*

Those who will not take up the process of Kṛṣṇa consciousness may sit silently in meditation and in this way stop all their nonsensical activity. But those who are advanced in Kṛṣṇa consciousness are constantly working for Kṛṣṇa. A mother tells only her bad child to sit down and do nothing. If a child can do nothing but disturb his mother, the mother says, "My dear child, just sit down here and keep quiet." But if the child can work nicely, the mother says, "My dear child, will you please help me do this? Will you go over there and do that?" Sitting still in one place is just for those who do not know how to work sensibly. As long as the child sits in one place, he does not raise havoc. Sitting still means negating nonsense; it is not positive activity. In negation, there is no life. Positive activities constitute life, and positive activity is the message of the *Bhagavad-gītā.* Spiritual life is not "Don't do this." Spiritual life is *"Do this!"* Of course, in order to act properly there are certain things that one must know not to do; therefore certain activities are forbidden. The whole *Bhagavad-gītā*, however, is "*do.*" Kṛṣṇa says, "Fight for Me." At the beginning of the *Bhagavad-gītā*, when Arjuna told Kṛṣṇa, "I will not fight," Śrī Kṛṣṇa said,

kutas tvā kaśmalam idaṁ viṣame samupasthitam
anārya juṣṭam asvargyaṁ akīrti-karam arjuna

"My dear Arjuna, how have these impurities come upon you? They are not at all befitting a man who knows the value of life. They lead not to higher planets but to infamy." (Bg. 2.2) Kṛṣṇa directly tells Arjuna that he is speaking like a non-Āryan—that is, like one who does not know the true value of human life. So Kṛṣṇa consciousness does not mean sitting down idly.

Kṛṣṇa Himself does not sit down idly. All His pastimes are filled with activity. When we go to the spiritual world, we will see that Kṛṣṇa is always engaged in dancing, eating, and enjoying. He does not sit down to meditate. Is there any account of the *gopīs* meditating? Did Caitanya Mahāprabhu sit down to meditate? No, He was always chanting Hare Kṛṣṇa and dancing. The spirit soul is naturally active. How can we sit down silently and do nothing? It is not possible. Therefore, after Śrī Kṛṣṇa outlined the *sāṅkhya-yoga* system in the Sixth Chapter of the *Bhagavad-gītā*, Arjuna frankly said,

yo 'yaṁ yogas tvayā proktaḥ sāmyena madhusūdana
etasyāhaṁ na paśyāmi cañcalatvāt sthitiṁ sthirām

"O Madhusūdana, the system of *yoga* which You have summarized appears impractical and unendurable to me, for the mind is restless and unsteady." (Bg. 6.33) Although Arjuna was highly elevated and was Kṛṣṇa's intimate friend, he immediately refused to take up the *sāṅkhya-yoga* system. In essence, he said, "It is not possible for me." How could it have been possible? Arjuna was a warrior and a householder, and he wanted a kingdom. What time did he have for meditation? He flatly refused to practice this type of meditational *yoga*, saying that the mind is as difficult to control as the wind (Bg. 6.34). That is a fact. It is not possible to control the mind artificially; therefore we must engage the mind in Kṛṣṇa consciousness. Then it is controlled. If Arjuna found this process more difficult than controlling the wind, then what of us? After all, Arjuna was not an ordinary man. He was personally talking with the Supreme Lord, Śrī Kṛṣṇa, and he proclaimed the mind to be like a great wind. How can we control the wind? We can control the mind only by fixing it on Kṛṣṇa's lotus feet. That is the perfection of meditation.

No one really wants to sit down and meditate. Why should we? We're meant for positive activity, for recreation, for pleasure. In Kṛṣṇa consciousness, our recreation is dancing and chanting, and when we get tired, we take *prasādam.* Is dancing difficult? Is chanting difficult? We don't charge anything to dance in the temple. If you go to a ballroom, you have to pay to enter, but we do not charge. It is natural to enjoy music and dancing and palatable foods. These are our recreations, and this is our method of meditation. So this *yoga* system is not at all laborious. It is simply recreation, *su-sukham.* It is stated in the Ninth Chapter of the *Bhagavad-gītā* (9.2) that this *yoga* is *su-sukham*—very happy. "It is everlasting, and it is joyfully performed." It is natural, automatic, and spontaneous. It is our real life in the spiritual world.

In Vaikuṇṭha, the spiritual world, there is no anxiety. *Vaikuṇṭha* means "freedom from anxiety," and in Vaikuṇṭha the liberated souls are always dancing, chanting, and taking *prasādam.* There are no factories, hard work, or technical institutions. There is no need for these artificial things. The *Vedānta-sūtra* states, *ānandamayo 'bhyāsāt:* God is *ānandamaya*, full of bliss and pleasure. Since we are part and parcel of God, we also possess these same qualities. So the goal of our *yoga* process is to join with the supreme *ānandamaya*, Śrī Kṛṣṇa, to join His dance party. Then we will be actually happy.

On this earth we are trying to be happy artificially and are therefore frustrated. Once we are situated in Kṛṣṇa consciousness, we will revive our original position and become simply joyful. Since our actual nature is *ānandamaya,* blissful, we are always searching for happiness. In the cities we are inundated with advertisements. Restaurants, bars, nightclubs, and dance halls are always announcing, "Come on, here is *ānanda.* Here is pleasure." That is because everyone is searching for *ānanda,* pleasure. Our society for Kṛṣṇa consciousness is also announcing, "Here is *ānanda,*" but our standard of pleasure is very different. In any case, the goal—pleasure—is the same.

Most people are hunting for pleasure on the gross material platform. The more advanced search for pleasure in speculation, philosophy, poetry, or art. The *bhakti-yogī,* however, searches for pleasure on the transcendental platform, and that is his only business. Why are people working so hard all day? They are thinking, "Tonight I shall enjoy. Tonight I will associate with this girl or with my wife." Thus people are going to so much trouble to acquire a little pleasure. Pleasure is the ultimate goal, but unfortunately, under illusion, people do not know where real pleasure is to be found. Real pleasure exists eternally in the transcendental form of Kṛṣṇa.

Perhaps you have seen pictures of Kṛṣṇa, and if so, you have noticed that Kṛṣṇa is always jolly. If you join His society, you will also become jolly. Have you ever seen pictures of Kṛṣṇa working with a machine? Have you ever seen pictures of Kṛṣṇa smoking? No, He is *by nature* full of pleasure, and if you unfold yourself in that way, if you wholeheartedly take up the process of Kṛṣṇa consciousness, you will also find pleasure. Pleasure cannot be found artificially.

ānanda-cinmaya-rasa-pratibhāvitābhis
tābhir ya eva nija-rūpatayā kalābhiḥ
goloka eva nivasaty akhilātma-bhūto
govindam ādi-puruṣaṁ tam ahaṁ bhajāmi

"I worship Govinda, the primeval Lord, who resides in His own realm, Goloka, with Rādhā, who resembles His own spiritual figure and who embodies the ecstatic potency. Their companions are Her confidantes, who embody extensions of Her bodily form and who are imbued and permeated with ever-blissful spiritual *rasa*." (*Brahma-saṁhitā* 5.37)

The word *rasa* means "taste," or "mellow." We enjoy sweets or candy because of their taste. Everyone is trying to enjoy some taste, and we want to enjoy sex because there is some taste there. That is the *ādi-rasa*, or original taste. Material tastes are quickly finished; they last only a few minutes. You may take a piece of candy, taste it, and say, "Oh, that is very nice," but you have to taste another in order to continue the enjoyment. And soon you will say, "No, I don't want any more." So material taste is limited, but real taste, spiritual taste, is without end. Once you experience the spiritual taste, you cannot forgot it; it will go on increasing. *Ānandāmbudhi-vardhanam.* Caitanya Mahāprabhu says, "This taste is always increasing." Spiritual taste is like the ocean in the sense that it is very great. The Pacific Ocean is always tossing, but it is not increasing. By God's order, the ocean does not extend beyond its limit, and if it extends, there is havoc. Lord Caitanya Mahāprabhu says that there is another ocean, an ocean of transcendental bliss, an ocean that is always increasing. *Ānandāmbudhi-vardhanaṁ prati-padaṁ pūrṇāmṛtāsvādanaṁ/ sarvātma-snapanaṁ paraṁ vijayate śrī-kṛṣṇa-saṅkīrtanam.* By chanting Hare Kṛṣṇa, our pleasure potency increases more and more.

Those who have realized Śrī Kṛṣṇa are always living in Vṛndāvana, Vaikuṇṭha. Although a devotee may seem to be living in some place far from Vṛndāvana, he is always living in Vṛndāvana, because he knows that Kṛṣṇa is present everywhere, even within the atom. The Supreme Lord is bigger than the biggest and smaller than the smallest. Once we are fully realized and established in Kṛṣṇa consciousness, we never lose sight of Kṛṣṇa, and our bliss is always increasing. This is the true *yoga* system, *bhakti-yoga*, as expounded by Lord Śrī Kṛṣṇa Himself in the *Bhagavad-gītā*.

2

Mastering the Mind and Senses

yaṁ sannyāsam iti prāhur yogaṁ taṁ viddhi pāṇḍava
na hy asannyasta-saṅkalpo yogī bhavati kaścana

"What is called renunciation you should know to be the same as *yoga*, or linking oneself with the Supreme, O son of Pāṇḍu, for one can never become a *yogī* unless he renounces the desire for sense gratification." (Bg. 6.2) This is the real purpose of the practice of *yoga*. The word *yoga* means "to join." Although we are naturally part and parcel of the Supreme, in our conditioned state we are now separated. Because of our separation, we are reluctant to understand God and to speak of our relationship with Him and are even inclined to think of such discussion as a waste of time. In a church or in a Kṛṣṇa consciousness temple, we speak of God, but people in general are not very interested. They think it is a waste of time, a kind of recreation in the name of spiritual advancement, and they believe that this time could be better used to earn money or enjoy themselves in a nightclub or restaurant.

Therefore, it is due to sense enjoyment that we are not attracted to God, and so it is said that those who are addicted to sense enjoyment cannot become *yogīs*—that is, they are not eligible to participate in the *yoga* system. One cannot advance in any *yoga* system if he partakes in sense gratification and then sits down to try to meditate. This is just a colossal hoax. Such contradictory activity has no meaning. First of all, *yoga* means controlling the senses—*yama-niyama.* There are eight stages of *yoga—yama, niyama, āsana, prāṇāyāma, pratyāhāra, dhāraṇā, dhyāna,* and *samādhi.*

In the Sixth Chapter of the *Bhagavad-gītā,* in which the Lord speaks of the *sāṅkhya-yoga* system, He states from the very beginning that one cannot become a *yogī* unless he renounces the desire for sense gratification. Therefore, if one indulges his senses, he cannot be accepted as a *yogī*. *Yoga* demands strict celibacy. In the *yoga* system, there is no sex life. If one indulges in sex, he cannot be a *yogī*. Many so-called *yogīs* come from India to America and say, "Yes, you can do whatever you like. You can have as much sex as you like. Just meditate. I will give you some *mantra*, and you will give me some money." This is all nonsense. According to the authoritative statements of Śrī Kṛṣṇa, one cannot become a *yogī* unless he renounces the desire for sense gratification. This is explicitly stated as the first condition for *yoga* practice.

ārurukṣor muner yogaṁ karma kāraṇam ucyate
yogārūḍhasya tasyaiva śamaḥ kāraṇam ucyate

"For one who is a neophyte in the eightfold *yoga* system, work is said to be the means, and for one who has already attained to *yoga*, cessation of all material activities is said to be the means." (Bg. 6.3) According to this verse, there are those who are attempting to reach the perfectional stage and those who have already attained that stage. As long as one is not situated on the perfectional platform, he must engage in so many activities. In the West, there are many *yoga* societies attempting to practice the *āsana* system, and therefore they practice sitting in different postures. That may help, but it is only a process by which one can attain the real platform. The real *yoga* system, in its perfectional stage, is far different from these bodily gymnastics.

It is important to understand, however, that from the beginning a Kṛṣṇa conscious person is situated on the platform of meditation because he is always thinking of Kṛṣṇa. Being constantly engaged in the service of Kṛṣṇa, he is considered to have ceased all material activities.

yadā hi nendriyārtheṣu na karmasv anuṣajjate
sarva-saṅkalpa-sannyāsī yogārūḍhas tadocyate

"A person is said to have attained to *yoga* when, having renounced all material desires, he neither acts for sense gratification nor engages in fruitive activities." (Bg. 6.4) This is actually the perfectional stage of *yoga*, and one who has attained this stage is said to have attained to *yoga*. This is to say that he has linked himself with the supreme whole. If a part is disconnected from a machine, it serves no function, but as soon as it is properly attached to the machine, it works properly and carries out its different functions. That is the meaning of *yoga*—joining with the supreme whole, serving in conjunction with the total machine. Presently we are disconnected, and our material, fruitive activities are simply a waste of time. One who engages in such activity is described in the *Bhagavad-gītā* as a *mūḍha*—that is, a rascal. Although one may earn thousands of dollars daily and be an important businessman, he is described in the *Bhagavad-gītā* as a *mūḍha*, rascal, because he is just wasting his time in eating, sleeping, defending, and mating.

People do not stop to consider that they are actually working very hard for nothing. One who earns millions of dollars cannot really eat much more than a man who makes ten dollars. A man who earns millions of dollars cannot mate with millions of women. That is not within his power. His mating power is the same as one who earns ten dollars, just as his power of eating is the same. This is to say that our power of enjoyment is limited. One should therefore think, "My enjoyment is the same as that of the man who is earning ten dollars daily. So why am I working so hard to earn millions of dollars? Why am I wasting my energy? I should engage my time and energy in understanding God. That is the purpose of life." If one has no economic problems, he has sufficient time to understand Kṛṣṇa consciousness. If he wastes this precious time, he is called a *mūḍha*, a rascal or an ass.

According to the preceding verse, a person is said to have attained *yoga* when he has renounced all material desires. Once we are situated perfectly in *yoga*, we are satisfied. We no longer experience material desires. We no longer act for sense gratification or engage in fruitive activity. When we speak of "fruitive activity," we refer to activities carried out for the purpose of sense gratification. That is, we are earning money in order to gratify our senses. If one is virtuous, he engages in pious activities—he donates money to charities, opens hospitals, schools, etc. Although these are certainly virtuous activities, they are ultimately meant for sense gratification. How is this? If I donate to an educational institution, for instance, I will receive good educational facilities and will become highly educated in my next life. Being thus educated, I will attain a good position and will acquire a good amount of money. Then how will I utilize this money? For sense gratification. Thus these virtuous and fruitive activities form a kind of cycle.

We often hear the expression "a better standard of living," but what does this mean? It is said that the standard of living in America is superior to that in India, but in both countries there is eating, sleeping, defending, and mating. Of course, in America the quality of food may be better, but the eating process is there. A superior standard of living does not mean superior spiritual realization. It just means better eating, sleeping, mating, and defending. This is called fruitive activity, and it is based on sense gratification.

Yoga has nothing to do with sense gratification or fruitive activity. *Yoga* means connecting with the Supreme. Dhruva Mahārāja underwent severe austerities in order to see God, and when he finally saw God, he said, *svāmin kṛtārtho 'smi varaṁ na yāce:* "My dear Lord, I am now fully satisfied. I am not asking for anything more. I do not want any further benediction from You." Why didn't Dhruva Mahārāja ask for benedictions? What is a benediction? Generally, *benediction* means receiving a great kingdom, a beautiful wife, palatable food, and so forth, but when one is actually connected with God, he does not want such benedictions. He is fully satisfied.

Actually, Dhruva Mahārāja initially searched for God in order to attain his father's kingdom. Dhruva Mahārāja's mother was rejected by his father, and his stepmother resented his sitting on his father's lap. Indeed, she forbade him to sit on his father's lap because Dhruva Mahārāja was not born from her womb. Although only five years old, Dhruva Mahārāja was a *kṣatriya*, and he took this as a great insult. Going to his own mother, he said, "Mother, my stepmother has insulted me by forbidding me to sit on my father's lap."

Dhruva Mahārāja then started to cry, and his mother said, "My dear boy, what can I do? Your father loves your stepmother more than he loves me. I can do nothing."

Dhruva Mahārāja then said, "But I want my father's kingdom. Tell me how I can get it."

"My dear boy," his mother said, "if Kṛṣṇa, God, blesses you, you can get it."

"Where is God?" Dhruva Mahārāja asked.

"Oh, it is said that God is in the forest," his mother said. "Great sages go to the forest to search for God."

Hearing this, Dhruva Mahārāja went directly to the forest and began to perform severe penances. Finally he saw God, and when he saw Him, he no longer desired his father's kingdom. Instead, he said, "My dear Lord, I was searching for some pebbles, but instead I have found valuable jewels. I no longer care for my father's kingdom. Now I am fully satisfied." When one is actually connected with God, he is totally satisfied. His satisfaction is infinitely greater than so-called enjoyment in this material world. That is the satisfaction resulting from God realization, and that is the perfection of *yoga.*

When a person is fully engaged in the transcendental loving service of the Lord, he is pleased in himself, and thus he is no longer engaged in sense gratification or in fruitive activities. Otherwise, one must be engaged in sense gratification, since one cannot live without engagement. It is impossible to cease all activity. As stated before, it is our nature as living entities to act. It is said, "An idle mind is the devil's workshop." If we have no Kṛṣṇa conscious engagement, we will engage in sense gratification or fruitive activity. If a child is not trained or educated, he becomes spoiled. If one does not practice the *yoga* system, if he does not attempt to control his senses by the *yoga* process, he will engage his senses in their own gratification. When one is gratifying his senses, there is no question of practicing *yoga.*

Without Kṛṣṇa consciousness, one must be always seeking self-centered or extended selfish activities. But a Kṛṣṇa conscious person can do everything for the satisfaction of Kṛṣṇa and thereby be perfectly detached from sense gratification. One who has not realized Kṛṣṇa must mechanically try to escape material desires before being elevated to the top rung of the *yoga* ladder.

One may compare the *yoga* system to a ladder. One *yogī* may be situated on the fifth step, another *yogī* may be on the fiftieth step, and yet another may be on the five-hundredth step. The purpose, of course, is to reach the top. Although the entire ladder may be called the *yoga* system, one who is on the fifth step is not equal to one who is higher up. In the *Bhagavad-gītā*, Śrī Kṛṣṇa delineates a number of *yoga* systems—*karma-yoga*, *jñāna-yoga*, *dhyāna-yoga*, and *bhakti-yoga*. All of these systems are connected with God, Kṛṣṇa, just as the entire ladder is connected to the topmost floor. This is not to say that everyone practicing the *yoga* system is situated on the topmost floor; only he who is in full Kṛṣṇa consciousness is so situated. Others are situated on different steps of the *yoga* ladder.

uddhared ātmanātmānaṁ nātmānam avasādayet
ātmaiva hy ātmano bandhur ātmaiva ripur ātmanaḥ

"A man must elevate himself by his own mind, not degrade himself. The mind is the friend of the conditioned soul, and his enemy as well." (Bg. 6.5) The word *ātmā* denotes body, mind, and soul, depending on different circumstances. In the *yoga* system, the mind and the conditioned soul are especially important. Since the mind is the central point of *yoga* practice, *ātmā* refers here to the mind. The purpose of the *yoga* system is to control the mind and to draw it away from attachment to sense objects. It is stressed herein that the mind must be so trained that it can deliver the conditioned soul from the mire of nescience.

In the *aṣṭāṅga-yoga* system, the eight practices—*dhyāna*, *dhāraṇā*, etc.—are meant for controlling the mind. Śrī Kṛṣṇa explicitly states that a man must utilize his mind to elevate himself. Unless one can control the mind, there is no question of elevation. The body is like a chariot, and the mind is the driver. If you tell your driver, "Please take me to the Kṛṣṇa temple," the driver will take you there, but if you tell him, "Please take me to that liquor house," you will go there. It is the driver's business to take you wherever you like. If you can control the driver, he will take you where you should go, but if not, he will ultimately take you wherever he likes. If you have no control over your driver, your driver is your enemy, but if he acts according to your orders, he is your friend.

The *yoga* system is meant to control the mind in such a way that the mind will act as your friend. Sometimes the mind acts as a friend and sometimes as an enemy. Because we are part and parcel of the Supreme, who has infinite independence, we have minute, or finite, independence. It is the mind that is controlling that independence, and therefore he may take us to either the Kṛṣṇa temple or some nightclub.

It is the purpose of the Kṛṣṇa consciousness movement to fix the mind on Kṛṣṇa. When the mind is so fixed, he cannot do anything but act as our friend. He has no scope to act any other way. As soon as Kṛṣṇa is seated in the mind, there is light, just as when the sun is in the sky, darkness is vanquished. Kṛṣṇa is just like the sun, and when He is present there is no scope for darkness. If we keep Kṛṣṇa on our mind, the darkness of *māyā* will never be able to enter. Keeping the mind fixed on Kṛṣṇa is the perfection of *yoga.* If the mind is strongly fixed on the Supreme, it will not allow any nonsense to enter, and there will be no falldown. If the mind is strong, the driver is strong, and we may go wherever we may desire. The entire *yoga* system is meant to make the mind strong, to make it incapable of deviating from the Supreme.

Sa vai manaḥ kṛṣṇa-padāravindayoḥ. One should fix his mind on Kṛṣṇa, just as Ambarīṣa Mahārāja did when he had a fight with a great *aṣṭāṅga-yogī* named Durvāsā Muni. Since Ambarīṣa Mahārāja was a householder, he was a pounds-shillings man. This means that he had to take into account pounds, shillings, and sixpence, or dollars and cents. Apart from being a householder, Mahārāja Ambarīṣa was also a great king and devotee. Durvāsā Muni was a great *yogī* who happened to be very envious of Mahārāja Ambarīṣa. Durvāsā Muni was thinking, "I am a great *yogī,* and I can travel in space. This man is an ordinary king, and he does not possess such yogic powers. Still, people pay him more honor. Why is this? I will teach him a good lesson." Durvāsā Muni then proceeded to pick a quarrel with Mahārāja Ambarīṣa, but because the king was always thinking of Kṛṣṇa, he managed to defeat this great *yogī.* Durvāsā Muni was consequently directed by Nārāyaṇa to take shelter at the feet of Mahārāja Ambarīṣa. Durvāsā Muni was such a perfect *yogī* that within a year he could travel throughout the material universe and also penetrate the spiritual universe. Indeed, he went directly to the abode of God, Vaikuṇṭha, and saw the Personality of Godhead Himself. Yet Durvāsā Muni was so weak that he had to return to earth and fall at the feet of Mahārāja Ambarīṣa. Mahārāja Ambarīṣa was an ordinary king, but his one great qualification was that he was always thinking of Kṛṣṇa. Thus his mind was always controlled, and he was situated at the highest perfectional level of *yoga.* We also can very easily control the mind by keeping it fixed on the lotus feet of Kṛṣṇa within. Simply by thinking of Kṛṣṇa, we become victorious conquerors, topmost *yogīs.*

Yoga indriya-saṁyamaḥ. The *yoga* system is meant for controlling the senses, and since the mind is above the senses, if we can control the mind, our senses are automatically controlled. The tongue may want to eat something improper, but if the mind is strong, it can say, "No. You cannot eat this. You can only eat *kṛṣṇa-prasādam.*" In this way the tongue, as well as all the other senses, can be controlled by the mind. *Indriyāṇi parāṇy āhur indriyebhyaḥ paraṁ manaḥ.* The material body consists of the senses, and consequently the body's activities are sensual activities. However, above the senses is the mind, and above the mind is the intelligence, and above the intelligence is the spirit soul. If one is on the spiritual platform, his intelligence, mind, and senses are all spiritualized. The purpose of the Kṛṣṇa consciousness process is to actualize the spiritualization of the senses, mind, and intelligence. The spirit soul is superior to all, but because he is sleeping, he has given power of attorney to the fickle mind. However, when the soul is awakened, he is once again master, and the servile mind cannot act improperly. Once we are awakened in Kṛṣṇa consciousness, the intelligence, mind, and senses cannot act nonsensically. They must act in accordance with the dictations of the spirit soul. That is spiritualization and purification. *Hṛṣīkeṇa hṛṣīkeśa-sevanaṁ bhaktir ucyate.* We must serve the master of the senses with the senses. The Supreme Lord is called Hṛṣīkeśa, which means that He is the original controller of the senses, just as a king is the original controller of all the activities of a state, and the citizens are secondary controllers.

Bhakti means acting spiritually in accordance with the desires of Hṛṣīkeśa. How can we act? Since we must act with our senses, we must spiritualize our senses in order to act properly. As stated before, sitting in silent meditation means stopping undesirable activity, but acting in Kṛṣṇa consciousness is transcendental. The cessation of nonsensical action is not in itself perfection. We must *act* perfectly. Unless we train our senses to act in accordance with the desires of Hṛṣīkeśa, the master of the senses, our senses will again engage in undesirable activities, and we will fall down. Therefore we must engage the senses in action for Kṛṣṇa and in this way remain firmly fixed in Kṛṣṇa consciousness.

In material existence one is subjected to the influence of the mind and the senses. In fact, the pure soul is entangled in the material world because the mind is involved with the false ego, which desires to lord it over material nature. Therefore, the mind should be trained so that it will not be attracted by the glitter of material nature, and in this way the conditioned soul may be saved. One should not degrade oneself by attraction to sense objects. The more one is attracted by sense objects, the more one becomes entangled in material existence. The best way to disentangle oneself is to always engage the mind in Kṛṣṇa consciousness. The word *hi* in verse 5, Chapter Six (*Bhagavad-gītā*), is used to emphasize this point—namely, that one *must* do this. It is also said,

mana eva manuṣyāṇāṁ kāraṇaṁ bandha-mokṣayoḥ
bandhāya viṣayāsaṅgo muktyai nirviṣayaṁ manaḥ

"For man, mind is the cause of bondage and mind is the cause of liberation. Mind absorbed in sense objects is the cause of bondage, and mind detached from the sense objects is the cause of liberation." (*Amṛta-bindu Upaniṣad* 2) The mind which is always engaged in Kṛṣṇa consciousness is the cause of supreme liberation. When the mind is thus engaged in Kṛṣṇa consciousness, there is no chance of its being engaged in *māyā* consciousness. In Kṛṣṇa consciousness, we remain in the sunlight, and there is no chance of our being obscured by darkness.

Because we have freedom, or liberty, we can stay within a dark room or go out into the broad daylight. That is our choice. Darkness can be eradicated by light, but light cannot be covered by darkness. If we are in a dark room and someone brings in a lamp, the darkness is vanquished. But we cannot take darkness into the sunlight. It is not possible. The darkness will simply fade away. *Kṛṣṇa sūrya-sama māyā haya andhakāra.*

Kṛṣṇa is like sunlight, and *māyā* is like darkness. So how can darkness exist in sunlight? If we always keep ourselves in the sunlight, darkness will fail to act upon us. This is the whole philosophy of Kṛṣṇa consciousness: always engage in Kṛṣṇa conscious activities, and *māyā* will be dissipated, just as darkness is dissipated when there is light. This is stated in *Śrīmad-Bhāgavatam* (1.7.4):

bhakti-yogena manasi samyak praṇihite 'male
apaśyat puruṣaṁ pūrṇaṁ māyāṁ ca tad-apāśrayam

"When the sage Vyāsadeva, under the instruction of his spiritual master, Nārada, fixed his mind, perfectly engaging it by linking it in devotional service (*bhakti-yoga*) without any tinge of materialism, Vyāsadeva saw the Absolute Personality of Godhead along with His external energy, which was under full control."

The word *manasi* refers to the mind. When one is enlightened in *bhakti-yoga*, the mind becomes completely freed from all contamination (*samyak praṇihite 'male*). When Vyāsa saw the Supreme Personality of Godhead, he saw *māyā* in the background (*māyāṁ ca tad-apāśrayam*). Whenever there is light, there is also the possibility of darkness being present. That is, darkness is the other side of light, or darkness is under the shelter of light, just as if I hold my hand up to the light, the top part of my hand will be in light, and the bottom part will be shaded. In other words, one side is light and the other darkness. When Vyāsadeva saw Kṛṣṇa, the Supreme Lord, he also saw *māyā*, darkness, under His shelter.

And what is this *māyā*? This is explained in the next verse of *Śrīmad-Bhāgavatam* (1.7.5):

yayā sammohito jīva ātmānaṁ tri-guṇātmakam
paro 'pi manute 'narthaṁ tat-kṛtaṁ cābhipadyate

"Due to the external energy, the living entity, although transcendental to the three modes of material nature, thinks of himself as a material product and thus undergoes the reactions of material miseries." Thus the illusory energy has temporarily covered the conditioned souls. And who are these conditioned souls? Although finite, the conditioned spirit souls are as full of light as Kṛṣṇa. The problem is that the conditioned soul identifies himself with this material world. This is called illusion, false identification with matter. Although the individual spirit soul is transcendental, he engages in improper activities under the dictation of *māyā,* and this brings about his conditioning or false identification. This is very elaborately explained in the Seventh Chapter, First Canto, of *Śrīmad-Bhāgavatam.*

In conclusion, our actual position is that of spiritual sparks, full of light. Now we are temporarily covered by this illusory energy, *māyā,* which is dictating to us. Acting under the influence of *māyā,* we are becoming more and more entangled in the material energy. The *yoga* system is meant to disentangle us, and the perfection of *yoga* is Kṛṣṇa consciousness. Thus Kṛṣṇa consciousness is the most effective means by which we can disentangle ourselves from the influence of the material energy.

3

Learning How to See God

bandhur ātmātmanas tasya yenātmaivātmanā jitaḥ
anātmanas tu śatrutve vartetātmaiva śatru-vat

"For him who has conquered the mind, the mind is the best of friends, but for one who has failed to do so, his mind will remain the greatest enemy." (Bg. 6.6)

The purpose of *yoga* is to make the mind into a friend. In material contact, the mind is in a kind of drunken condition. As stated in *Caitanya-caritāmṛta* (*Madhya* 20.117),

kṛṣṇa bhuli' sei jīva—anādi-bahirmukha
ataeva māyā tāre deya saṁsāra-duḥkha

"Forgetting Kṛṣṇa, the living entity has been attracted by the Lord's external feature from time immemorial. Therefore the illusory energy (*māyā*) gives him all kinds of misery in his material existence." The living entity is constitutionally spirit soul, part and parcel of the Supreme Lord. As soon as the mind is contaminated, the living entity, because he has a little independence, rebels. In this state, the mind dictates, "Why should I serve Kṛṣṇa? I am God." Thus one labors under a false impression, and his life is spoiled. We try to conquer many things—even empires—but if we fail to conquer the mind, we are failures even if we manage to conquer an empire. Even though emperors, we will have within us our greatest enemy—our own mind.

jitātmanaḥ praśāntasya paramātmā samāhitaḥ
śītoṣṇa-sukha-duḥkheṣu tathā mānāpamānayoḥ

"For one who has conquered the mind, the Supersoul is already reached, for he has attained tranquillity. To such a man happiness and distress, heat and cold, honor and dishonor are all the same." (Bg. 6.7)

Actually, every living entity is intended to abide by the dictation of the Supreme Personality of Godhead, who is seated in everyone's heart as the Paramātmā. When the mind is misled by the external, illusory energy, one becomes entangled in material activities. Therefore, as soon as one's mind is controlled through one of the *yoga* systems, one should be considered to have already reached the destination. One has to abide by superior dictation. When one's mind is fixed on the superior nature, one has no alternative but to follow the dictation of the Supreme. The mind must admit some superior dictation and follow it. When the mind is controlled, one automatically follows the dictation of the Paramātmā, or Supersoul. Because this transcendental position is at once achieved by one who is in Kṛṣṇa consciousness, the devotee of the Lord is unaffected by the dualities of material existence—distress and happiness, cold and heat, etc. This state is called *samādhi,* or absorption in the Supreme.

jñāna-vijñāna-tṛptātmā kūṭa-stho vijitendriyaḥ
yukta ity ucyate yogī sama-loṣṭrāśma-kāñcanaḥ

"A person is said to be established in self-realization and is called a *yogī* [or mystic] when he is fully satisfied by virtue of acquired knowledge and realization. Such a person is situated in transcendence and is self-controlled. He sees everything—whether it be pebbles, stones, or gold—as the same." (Bg. 6.8)

Book knowledge without realization of the Supreme Truth is useless. This is stated as follows:

ataḥ śrī-kṛṣṇa-nāmādi na bhaved grāhyam indriyaiḥ
sevonmukhe hi jihvādau svayam eva sphuraty adaḥ

"No one can understand the transcendental nature of the name, form, qualities, and pastimes of Śrī Kṛṣṇa through his materially contaminated senses. Only when one becomes spiritually saturated by transcendental service to the Lord are the transcendental name, form, qualities, and pastimes of the Lord revealed to him." (*Bhakti-rasāmṛta-sindhu* 1.2.234)

There are men in the modes of goodness, passion, and ignorance, and to reclaim all these conditioned souls, there are eighteen *Purāṇas*. Six *Purāṇas* are meant for persons in the mode of goodness, six for those in the mode of passion, and six for those in the mode of ignorance. The *Padma Purāṇa* is written for those in the mode of goodness. Because there are many different types of men, there are many different Vedic rituals. In the Vedic literatures there are descriptions of rituals and ceremonies in which a goat may be sacrificed in the presence of the goddess Kālī. This is described in the *Mārkaṇḍeya Purāṇa*, but this *Purāṇa* is meant for the instruction of those in the mode of ignorance.

It is very difficult for one to give up his attachments all at once. If one is addicted to meat-eating and is suddenly told that he must not eat meat, he cannot do so. If one is attached to drinking liquor and is suddenly told that liquor is no good, he cannot accept this advice. Therefore, in the *Purāṇas* we find certain instructions that say in essence, "All right, if you want to eat meat, just worship the goddess Kālī and sacrifice a goat for her. Only then can you eat meat. You cannot eat meat just by purchasing it from the butcher shop. No, there must be sacrifice or restriction." In order to sacrifice a goat to the goddess Kālī, one must make arrangements for a certain date and utilize certain paraphernalia. That type of *pūjā*, or worship, is allowed on the night of the dark moon, which means once a month. There are also certain *mantras* to be chanted when the goat is sacrificed. The goat is told, "Your life is being sacrificed before the goddess Kālī; you will therefore be immediately promoted to the human form." Generally, in order to attain the human form, a living entity has to pass through many species of life on the evolutionary scale, but if a goat is sacrificed to the goddess Kālī, he is immediately promoted to the human form. The *mantra* also says, "You have the right to kill this man who is sacrificing you." The word *māṁsa* indicates that in his next birth the goat will eat the flesh of the man who is presently sacrificing him. This in itself should bring the goat-eater to his senses. He should consider, "Why am I eating this flesh? Why am I doing this? I'll have to repay with my own flesh in another life." The whole idea is to discourage one from eating meat.

Thus, because there are different types of men, there are eighteen *Purāṇas* to guide them. The Vedic literatures are meant to redeem all men, not just a few. It is not that those who are meat-eaters or drunkards are rejected. A doctor accepts all patients, and he prescribes different medicines according to the disease. It is not that he gives the same medicine for all diseases or that he treats just one disease. No, he offers a specific type of medicine to whoever comes, and the patient receives gradual treatment. However, the sattvic *Purāṇas* like the *Padma Purāṇa* are meant for those in the mode of goodness, for those who immediately are capable of worshiping the Supreme Personality of Godhead.

In the *Brahma-saṁhitā* it is stated, *īśvaraḥ paramaḥ kṛṣṇaḥ sac-cid-ānanda-vigrahaḥ:* "The supreme controller is Kṛṣṇa, who has an eternal, blissful, spiritual body." This is the Vedic pronouncement, and we thus accept Śrī Kṛṣṇa as the Supreme Lord. Those who are in the modes of passion and ignorance attempt to imagine the form of God, and when they are confused, they say, "Oh, there is no personal God. God is impersonal, or void." This is just the result of frustration. Actually, God has His form. Why not? According to the *Vedānta-sūtra*, *janmādy asya yataḥ:* "The Supreme Absolute Truth is He from whom everything emanates." It is easy to see that we have different types of bodies, different types of forms. We must consider where these forms are coming from. Where have these forms originated? We have to use a little common sense. If God is not a person, how can His sons be persons? If your father is just a void, if he is not a person, how can you be a person? If your father has no form, how can you have form? So it is not very difficult to understand that God must be a person with form; it is just common sense. Unfortunately, because people are frustrated, they conclude that because our material forms are temporary and troublesome, God must be formless.

The *Brahma-saṁhitā* specifically states that this conception is a mistake. *Īśvaraḥ paramaḥ kṛṣṇaḥ sac-cid-ānanda-vigrahaḥ.* God has form, but His form is *sac-cid-ānanda-vigraha. Sat* means "eternal," *cit* means "knowledge," and *ānanda* means "pleasure." God has form, but His form is eternal and is full of knowledge and pleasure. We cannot compare His form to our form. Our form is neither eternal, full of pleasure, nor full of knowledge; therefore God's form is different.

As soon as we speak of form, we think that this form must be like ours, and we therefore conclude that the eternal, all-knowing, and all-blissful God must be without form. This is not knowledge but the result of imperfect speculation. According to the *Padma Purāṇa, ataḥ śrī-kṛṣṇa-nāmādi na bhaved grāhyam indriyaiḥ:* "One cannot understand the form, name, qualities, or paraphernalia of God with one's material senses." Since our senses are imperfect, we cannot speculate on Him who is supremely perfect. That is not possible.

Then how is it possible to understand Him? *Sevonmukhe hi jihvādau.* By training and purifying our senses, we may come to understand and see God. Presently we are attempting to understand God with impure, imperfect senses. It is like someone with cataracts trying to see. Just because one has cataracts, he should not conclude that there is nothing to be seen. Similarly, we cannot presently conceive of God's form, but once our "cataracts" are removed, we can see Him. According to the *Brahma-saṁhitā, premāñjana-cchurita-bhakti-vilocanena santaḥ sadaiva hṛdayeṣu vilokayanti:* "The devotees whose eyes are anointed with the ointment of love of God can see God within their hearts twenty-four hours a day." Purification of the senses is what is required; then we can understand the name, form, qualities, and pastimes of God. Then we'll be able to see God everywhere and in everything.

These matters are discussed thoroughly in the Vedic literatures. For instance, it is said that although God has no hands or legs He can accept whatever we offer (*apāṇi-pādo javano gṛhītā*). It is also stated that although God has neither eyes nor ears He can see and hear everything. These are apparent contradictions, but they are meant to teach us an important lesson. When we speak of seeing, we think of material vision. Due to our material conception, we think that the eyes of God must be like ours. Therefore, in order to remove these material conceptions, the Vedic literatures say that God has no hands, legs, eyes, ears, etc. God has eyes, but His vision is infinite. He can see in darkness, and He can see everywhere at once; therefore He has different eyes. Similarly, God has ears and can hear. He may be in His kingdom, millions and millions of miles away, but He can hear us whispering because He is sitting within. We cannot avoid God's seeing, hearing, or touching.

patraṁ puṣpaṁ phalaṁ toyaṁ yo me bhaktyā prayacchati
tad ahaṁ bhakty-upahṛtam aśnāmi prayatātmanaḥ

"If one offers Me with love and devotion a leaf, a flower, a fruit, or water, I will accept it." (Bg. 9.26) If God does not have senses, how can He accept and eat the offerings that are presented to Him? According to ritual, we are offering Kṛṣṇa food daily, and we can see that the taste of this food is immediately changed. This is a practical example. God eats, but because He is full in Himself, He does not eat like us. If I offer you a plate of food, you will eat it, and it will be finished. God is not hungry, but He eats, and at the same time He leaves the food as it is, and thus it is transformed into *prasādam*, His mercy. *Pūrṇasya pūrṇam ādāya pūrṇam evāvaśiṣyate.* God is full in Himself, and so even though He accepts all the food that we offer, the food remains as it is. He can eat with His eyes. As stated in *Brahma-saṁhitā, aṅgāni yasya sakalendriya-vṛttimanti:* "Every sense of the Lord's body has all the potencies of the other senses." Although we can see with our eyes, we cannot eat with our eyes. The senses of God, however, being infinite, are different. Simply by looking at the food that is offered to Him, He eats it.

We may not understand this at the present moment; therefore the *Padma Purāṇa* states that when one becomes spiritually saturated by rendering transcendental service to the Lord, the transcendental name, form, qualities, and pastimes of the Lord are revealed. We cannot understand God by our own endeavor, but out of mercy God reveals Himself to us. If it is night and you want to see the sun, you will have to wait for the sun to appear in the morning. You cannot go outside with a big torch and say, "Come on, I will show you the sunlight." In the morning, when the sun rises of its own will, we can see it. Because our senses are imperfect, we cannot see God by our own endeavor. We have to purify our senses and wait for the time when God will be pleased to reveal Himself to us. That is the process. We cannot challenge God. We cannot say, "O my dear God, my dear Kṛṣṇa. Please come. I want to see You." No, God is not our order-supplier. He is not our servant. When He is pleased, we will see Him; therefore Kṛṣṇa consciousness is a process by which we can please God so that He will reveal Himself to us.

Because people cannot see God, they readily accept anyone who says, "I am God." Because people have no conception of God, they are eager to accept any rascal who comes along and proclaims himself to be God. People are fond of saying, "I am searching after the truth," but in order to search for the truth, we must know what the truth is. Otherwise, how can we search it out? If we want to purchase gold, we must at least theoretically know what gold is; otherwise we will be cheated. Similarly, because people have no conception of the truth or of God, they are being cheated by so many rascals who say, "I am God." Indeed, in a society of rascals, one rascal will accept another rascal as God. But all this has nothing to do with actually seeing God. One has to qualify himself to see and understand God, and that process of qualification is called Kṛṣṇa consciousness. *Sevonmukhe hi jihvādau svayam eva sphuraty adaḥ:* by engaging ourselves in God's service, we become qualified to see God. Otherwise it is not possible. We may be great scientists or scholars, but our mundane scholarship will not help us see God.

The *Bhagavad-gītā* is the science of Kṛṣṇa consciousness, and in order to understand Kṛṣṇa we must be fortunate enough to associate with a person who is in pure Kṛṣṇa consciousness, who possesses realized knowledge by the grace of Kṛṣṇa. We cannot understand the *Bhagavad-gītā* simply by acquiring an M.A., Ph.D., or whatever. The *Bhagavad-gītā* is a transcendental science, and we require different senses in order to understand it. We must purify our senses by rendering service to Kṛṣṇa, not by acquiring academic degrees. There are many Ph.D.'s, many scholars, who cannot understand Kṛṣṇa. Therefore Kṛṣṇa appears in the material world. Although He is unborn (*ajo 'pi sann avyayātmā*), He comes to reveal Himself to us.

Thus Kṛṣṇa is realized by the grace of Kṛṣṇa. We cannot understand Him through academic knowledge. We can understand Kṛṣṇa only by acquiring His grace. Once we acquire His grace, we can see Him, talk with Him—do whatever we desire. It is not that Kṛṣṇa is a void. He is a person, the Supreme Person, and we can have a relationship with Him. That is the Vedic injunction. *Nityo nityānāṁ cetanaś cetanānām:* "We are all eternal persons, and God is the supreme eternal person." Presently, because we are encaged within these bodies, we are experiencing birth and death, but actually we are beyond birth and death. We are eternal spirit souls, but according to our work and desires we are transmigrating from one body to another. It is explained in the Second Chapter of the *Bhagavad-gītā* (2.20),

> *na jāyate mriyate vā kadācin*
> *nāyaṁ bhūtvā bhavitā vā na bhūyaḥ*
> *ajo nityaḥ śāśvato 'yaṁ purāṇo*
> *na hanyate hanyamāne śarīre*

"For the soul there is neither birth nor death at any time. He has not come into being, does not come into being, and will not come into being. He is unborn, eternal, ever-existing, and primeval. He is not slain when the body is slain."

Just as God is eternal, we are also eternal, and when we establish our eternal relationship with the supreme, complete eternal, we realize our eternality. *Nityo nityānāṁ cetanaś cetanānām.* God is the supreme living entity among all living entities, the supreme eternal among all eternals. By Kṛṣṇa consciousness, by purification of the senses, this knowledge will be realized, and we will come to see God.

A Kṛṣṇa conscious person has realized knowledge, by the grace of Kṛṣṇa, because he is satisfied with pure devotional service. By realized knowledge, one becomes perfect. By transcendental knowledge one can remain steady in his convictions, but by mere academic knowledge one can be easily deluded and confused by apparent contradictions. It is the realized soul who is actually self-controlled, because he is surrendered to Kṛṣṇa. He is transcendental because he has nothing to do with mundane scholarship. For him, mundane scholarship and mental speculation, which may be as good as gold to others, are of no greater value than pebbles or stones.

Even one who is illiterate can realize God simply by engaging in submissive, transcendental loving service. God is not subject to any material condition. He is supreme spirit, and the process of realizing Him is also beyond material considerations. Therefore, one may be a very learned scholar and still not be able to understand God. One who is very poor should not think that he cannot realize God, nor should one who is very rich think that he can easily realize God. God may be understood by an uneducated person and misunderstood by one with great education. The understanding of God, like God Himself, is unconditional (*apratihata*).

In *Śrīmad-Bhāgavatam* (1.2.6) it is stated,

> *sa vai puṁsāṁ paro dharmo yato bhaktir adhokṣaje*
> *ahaituky apratihatā yayātmā suprasīdati*

"The supreme occupation (*dharma*) for all humanity is that by which men can attain to loving devotional service unto the transcendent Lord. Such devotional service must be unmotivated and uninterrupted to completely satisfy the self." Cultivation of love of God: that is the definition of first-class religion. Otherwise, there are various religious conceptions determined according to the three *guṇas*, or qualities, in the material world. We are not, however, concerned with analyzing these religious conceptions. From *Śrīmad-Bhāgavatam* we know that the purpose of religion is to understand God and to learn how to love God. That is the real purpose of any first-class religious system. If a religion does not teach love of God, it is useless. One may follow his religious principles very carefully, but if one does not possess love of God, his religion is null and void. According to *Śrīmad-Bhāgavatam* (1.2.6) real religion must be *ahaitukī* and *apratihatā:* without selfish motivation and without impediment. By practicing such a religion, we will become happy in all respects.

Sa vai puṁsāṁ paro dharmo yato bhaktir adhokṣaje. Another name for God is *adhokṣaja*, which means "one who cannot be seen by materialistic attempts." That is to say that God conquers all our attempts to see Him materially. The word *akṣaja* refers to experimental knowledge, and *adhaḥ* means "unreachable." So God cannot be reached through experimental knowledge. We have to learn to contact Him in a different way: through submissive hearing and the rendering of transcendental loving service.

True religion teaches causeless love of God. It does not say, "I love God because He supplies me nice objects for my sense gratification." That is not love. God is great, God is our eternal father, and it is our duty to love Him. There is no question of barter or exchange. We should not think, "Oh, God gives me my daily bread; therefore I love God." God gives daily bread even to the cats and dogs. Since He is the father of everyone, He is supplying everyone food. So loving God for daily bread is not love. Love is without reason. Even if God does not supply us our daily bread, we should love Him. That is true love. As Caitanya Mahāprabhu said,

āśliṣya vā pāda-ratāṁ pinaṣṭu mām
adarśanān marma-hatāṁ karotu vā
yathā tathā vā vidadhātu lampaṭo
mat-prāṇa-nāthas tu sa eva nāparaḥ

"I know no one but Kṛṣṇa as My Lord, and He shall remain so even if He handles Me roughly by His embrace or makes Me broken-hearted by not being present before Me. He is completely free to do anything and everything, for He is always My worshipful Lord, unconditionally." That is the sentiment of one who is established in pure love of God. When we attain that stage of love of God, we will find that everything is full of pleasure; God is full of pleasure, and we also are full of pleasure.

suhṛn-mitrāry-udāsīna-madhyastha-dveṣya-bandhuṣu
sādhuṣv api ca pāpeṣu sama-buddhir viśiṣyate

"A person is considered still further advanced when he regards honest well-wishers, affectionate benefactors, the neutral, mediators, the envious, friends and enemies, the pious and the sinners all with an equal mind." (Bg. 6.9) This is a sign of real spiritual advancement. In this material world we are considering people friends and enemies on the bodily platform—that is, on the basis of sense gratification. If someone gratifies our senses, he is our friend, and if he doesn't, he is our enemy. However, once we have realized God, or the Absolute Truth, there are no such material considerations.

In this material world, all conditioned souls are under illusion, in a diseased condition. A doctor treats all patients, and although a patient may be delirious and insult the doctor, the doctor does not refuse to treat him. He still administers the medicine that is required. As Lord Jesus Christ said, we should hate the sin, not the sinner. That is a very nice statement, because the sinner is under illusion. He is mad. If we hate him, how can we deliver him? Therefore, advanced devotees, those who are really servants of God, do not hate anyone. When Lord Jesus Christ was being crucified, he said, "My God, forgive them. They know not what they do." This is the proper attitude of an advanced devotee. He understands that the conditioned souls cannot be hated, because they have become mad due to their materialistic way of thinking. In the Kṛṣṇa consciousness movement there is no question of hating anyone. All are welcome to come and chant Hare Kṛṣṇa, take *kṛṣṇa-prasādam,* listen to the philosophy of the *Bhagavad-gītā,* and try to rectify their material, conditioned life. This is the essential program of Kṛṣṇa consciousness. Therefore, Lord Caitanya Mahāprabhu said, *yāre dekha, tāre kaha 'kṛṣṇa'-upadeśa:* "Whoever you meet, simply try to teach him Kṛṣṇa consciousness."

yogī yuñjīta satatam ātmānaṁ rahasi sthitaḥ
ekākī yata-cittātmā nirāśīr aparigrahaḥ

"A transcendentalist should always try to concentrate his mind on the Supreme Self. He should live alone in a secluded place and should always carefully control his mind. He should be free from desires and possessiveness." (Bg. 6.10)

Here in Chapter Six of the *Bhagavad-gītā* the Lord is teaching the principles of the *aṣṭāṅga-yoga* system, and now he begins His practical instruction by pointing out that a transcendentalist should always try to concentrate his mind on the Supreme Self. "The Supreme Self" refers to Kṛṣṇa, the Supreme Lord. As explained before (*nityo nityānāṁ cetanaś cetanānām*), God is the supreme eternal living entity, the Supreme Self. The purpose of the entire *yoga* system is to concentrate the mind on this Supreme Self. We are not the Supreme Self. That should be understood. The Supreme Self is God. This is *dvaita-vāda*—dualism—the understanding that God is different from me. He is supreme and I am subordinate. He is great and I am small. He is infinite and I am infinitesimal. This is the relationship between ourselves and God as we should understand it. Because we are infinitesimal, we should concentrate our mind on the infinite Supreme Self. In order to do this, we should live alone, and "living alone" means that we should not live with those who are not Kṛṣṇa conscious. This is a most important item in the practice of Kṛṣṇa consciousness. Living alone may mean living in a secluded place like a forest or a jungle, but in this age living in such a secluded place is very difficult. Therefore for us "secluded place" refers to that place where God consciousness is taught.

The transcendentalist should also carefully control his mind, and this means fixing the mind on the Supreme Self, or Kṛṣṇa. As explained before, Kṛṣṇa is just like the sun, and if the mind is fixed on Him, there is no question of darkness. If Kṛṣṇa is always on our minds, *māyā,* or illusion, can never enter. This is the process of concentration.

The transcendentalist should also be free from desires and feelings of possessiveness. People are materially diseased because they desire things and want to possess them. We hanker for that which we do not have, and we lament for that which we have lost. But one who is actually God conscious has no such feelings because he does not desire material possessions (*brahma-bhūtaḥ prasannātmā na śocati na kāṅkṣati*). He has only one desire—to serve Kṛṣṇa. It is not possible to give up desire, but it *is* possible to purify our desires. It is the nature of the living entity to have some desire, but in the conditioned state one's desire is contaminated. Conditioned, one thinks, "I desire to satisfy my senses by material possession." Purified desire is desire for Kṛṣṇa, and if we desire Kṛṣṇa, desires for material possessions will automatically vanish.

śucau deśe pratiṣṭhāpya sthiram āsanam ātmanaḥ
nāty-ucchritaṁ nāti-nīcaṁ cailājina-kuśottaram

tatraikāgraṁ manaḥ kṛtvā yata-cittendriya-kriyaḥ
upaviśyāsane yuñjyād yogam ātma-viśuddhaye

"To practice *yoga,* one should go to a secluded place and should lay *kuśa* grass on the ground and then cover it with a deerskin and a soft cloth. The seat should be neither too high nor too low and should be situated in a sacred place. The *yogī* should then sit on it very firmly and practice *yoga* by controlling his mind, senses, and activities and fixing the mind on one point." (Bg. 6.11–12) In these verses it is emphasized how and where one should sit. In the United States and other Western countries, there are many so-called *yoga* societies, but they do not practice *yoga* according to these prescriptions. "A sacred place" refers to a place of pilgrimage. In India, the *yogīs,* the transcendentalists or the devotees, all leave home and reside in sacred places such as Prayāga, Mathurā, Vṛndāvana, Hṛṣīkeśa, or Hardwar and in solitude practice *yoga* where sacred rivers like the Yamunā or the Ganges flow. So how is this possible in this age? How many people are prepared to go to such a sacred place? In order to earn one's livelihood, one has to live in a congested city; there is no question of residing in a sacred place. But for the practice of *yoga,* that is the first prerequisite.

Therefore in the *bhakti-yoga* system the temple is considered the sacred place. The temple is *nirguṇa*—transcendental. According to the *Vedas,* a city is in the mode of passion, a forest is in the mode of goodness, and a temple is transcendental. If you live in a city or town, you live in a place where passion is predominant, and if you want to escape this, you may go to a forest, a place of goodness. God's temple, however, is above passion and goodness; therefore the temple of Kṛṣṇa is the only secluded place for this age. In this age it is not possible to retreat to a forest; nor is it useful to make a show of practicing *yoga* in so-called *yoga* societies and at the same time engage in nonsense.

Therefore, in the *Bṛhan-nāradīya Purāṇa* it is said that in Kali-yuga, when people are generally short-lived, slow in spiritual realization, and always disturbed by various anxieties, the best means of spiritual realization is chanting the holy names of the Lord.

harer nāma harer nāma harer nāmaiva kevalam
kalau nāsty eva nāsty eva nāsty eva gatir anyathā

"In this age of quarrel and hypocrisy, the only means of deliverance is chanting the holy name of the Lord. There is no other way. There is no other way. There is no other way."

This is the solution, the grand gift of Caitanya Mahāprabhu. In this age, other *yoga* practices are not feasible, but this practice is so simple and universal that even a child can take to it.

4

Moderation in Yoga

In the Sixth Chapter of the *Bhagavad-gītā*, the system of *sāṅkhya-yoga*, which is the meditational *aṣṭāṅga-yoga* system, is emphasized. *Jñāna-yoga* emphasizes the philosophical process of analysis by which we determine what is Brahman and what is not Brahman. This process is known as the *neti neti* process, or "not this, not that." In the beginning of the *Vedānta-sūtra* it is stated, *janmādy asya yataḥ:* "The Supreme Brahman, the Absolute Truth, is He from whom everything emanates." This is a hint, and from this we must try to understand the nature of the Supreme Brahman, from whom everything is emanating. The nature of that Absolute Truth is explained in detail in *Śrīmad-Bhāgavatam.*

In the first verse of *Śrīmad-Bhāgavatam* it is stated,

oṁ namo bhagavate vāsudevāya
janmādy asya yato 'nvayād itarataś cārtheṣv abhijñaḥ svarāṭ
tene brahma hṛdā ya ādi-kavaye muhyanti yat sūrayaḥ
tejo-vāri-mṛdāṁ yathā vinimayo yatra tri-sargo 'mṛṣā
dhāmnā svena sadā nirasta-kuhakaṁ satyaṁ paraṁ dhīmahi

"O my Lord, Śrī Kṛṣṇa, son of Vasudeva, O all-pervading Personality of Godhead, I offer my respectful obeisances unto You. I meditate upon Lord Śrī Kṛṣṇa because He is the Absolute Truth and the primeval cause of all causes of the creation, sustenance, and destruction of the manifested universes. He is directly and indirectly conscious of all manifestations, and He is independent because there is no other cause beyond Him. It is He only who first imparted the Vedic knowledge unto the heart of Brahmājī, the original living being. By Him even the great sages and demigods are placed into illusion, as one is bewildered by the illusory representations of water seen in fire, or land seen on water. Only because of Him do the material universes, temporarily manifested by the reactions of the three modes of nature, appear factual, although they are unreal. I therefore meditate upon Him, Lord Śrī Kṛṣṇa, who is eternally existent in the transcendental abode. which is forever free from the illusory representations of the material world. I meditate upon Him, for He is the Absolute Truth."

Thus from the very beginning of *Śrīmad-Bhāgavatam* the Absolute Truth is proclaimed to be cognizant. He is not dead or void. And what is the nature of His cognizance? *Anvayād itarataś cārtheṣu:* "He is directly and indirectly cognizant of all manifestations." To a limited degree, each and every living entity is cognizant, but we are not completely cognizant. I may claim, "This is my head," but if someone asks me, "Do you know how many hairs are on your head?" I will not be able to reply. Of course, this kind of knowledge is not transcendental, but in *Śrīmad-Bhāgavatam* it is stated that the Supreme Absolute Truth knows everything, directly and indirectly. I may know that I am eating, but I do not know the intricacies of the eating process—exactly how my body is assimilating food, how the blood is passing through my veins, etc. I am cognizant that my body is functioning, but I do not know how these processes are working perfectly and all at once. This is because my knowledge is limited.

By definition, God is He who knows everything. He knows what is going on in every corner of His creation; therefore, from the very beginning *Śrīmad-Bhāgavatam* explains that the Supreme Truth, from whom everything is emanating, is supremely cognizant (*abhijñaḥ*). One may ask, "If the Absolute Truth is so powerful, wise, and cognizant, He must have attained this knowledge from some similar being." This is not the case. If He attains His knowledge from someone else, He is not God. He is independent (*svarāṭ*), and His knowledge is automatically there.

Śrīmad-Bhāgavatam is the supreme combination of both the *jñāna-* and *bhakti-yoga* systems because it analyzes in detail the nature of that Supreme Being, from whom everything is emanating. By the *jñāna-yoga* system, one attempts to understand the nature of the Absolute Truth in a philosophical way. In the *bhakti-yoga* system, the target is the same. The methodology, however, is somewhat different. Whereas the *jñānī* attempts to concentrate his mind philosophically on the Supreme, the *bhakta* simply engages himself in the service of the Supreme Lord, and the Lord reveals Himself. The *jñāna* method is called the ascending process, and the *bhakti* method is called the descending process. If we are in the darkness of night, we may attempt to see the sun by ascending in a powerful rocket. According to the descending process, however, we simply await the sunrise, and then we see the sun immediately.

Through the ascending process, we attempt to reach the Supreme through our own endeavor, through the process of induction. By induction, we may attempt to find out whether man is mortal by studying thousands of men, trying to see whether they are mortal or immortal. This, of course, will take a great deal of time, and at the end there will be no certainty. If, however, I accept from superior authority the fact that all men are mortal, my knowledge is complete and immediate. Thus it is stated in *Śrīmad-Bhāgavatam* (10.14.29), "My dear Lord, a person who has received a little favor from You can understand You very quickly. But those who are trying to understand You by the ascending process may go on speculating for millions of years and still never understand You."

By mental speculation, one is more likely simply to reach a point of frustration and confusion and conclude, "Oh, God is zero." But if God is zero, how are so many figures emanating from Him? As the *Vedānta-sūtra* says, *janmādy asya yataḥ:* "Everything is generated from the Supreme." Therefore the Supreme cannot be zero. We have to study how so many forms, an infinite number of living entities, are being generated from the Supreme. This is also explained in the *Vedānta-sūtra,* which is the study of ultimate knowledge. The word *veda* means "knowledge," and *anta* means "ultimate." Ultimate knowledge is knowledge of the Supreme Lord.

So how is it possible to understand the form of Kṛṣṇa? If it is stated that God does not have eyes, limbs, and senses like ours, how are we to understand His transcendental senses, His transcendental form? This is not possible by mental speculation. We simply have to serve Him, and then He will reveal Himself to us. As Kṛṣṇa Himself states in the Tenth Chapter of the *Bhagavad-gītā* (10.11),

> *teṣām evānukampārtham aham ajñāna-jaṁ tamaḥ*
> *nāśayāmy ātma-bhāva-stho jñāna-dīpena bhāsvatā*

"Out of compassion for My devotees, I, dwelling in their hearts, destroy with the shining lamp of knowledge the darkness born of ignorance." Kṛṣṇa is within us, and when we are sincerely searching for Him by the devotional process, He will reveal Himself.

Again, as Kṛṣṇa states in the Eighteenth Chapter of the *Bhagavad-gītā* (18.55),

> *bhaktyā mām abhijānāti yāvān yaś cāsmi tattvataḥ*
> *tato māṁ tattvato jñātvā viśate tad-anantaram*

"One can understand Me as I am, as the Supreme Personality of Godhead, only by devotional service. And when one is in full consciousness of Me by such devotion, he can enter into the kingdom of God." Thus God has to be understood by this process of *bhakti-yoga,* which is the process of *śravaṇaṁ kīrtanaṁ viṣṇoḥ*—hearing and chanting about Viṣṇu. This is the beginning of the *bhakti-yoga* process. If we but hear sincerely and submissively, we will understand. Kṛṣṇa will reveal Himself. *Śravaṇaṁ kīrtanaṁ viṣṇoḥ smaraṇaṁ pāda-sevanam arcanaṁ vandanaṁ dāsyam.* There are nine different processes in the *bhakti-yoga* system. By *vandanam,* we offer prayers, and that is also *bhakti. Śravaṇam* is hearing about Kṛṣṇa from the *Bhagavad-gītā, Śrīmad-Bhāgavatam,* and other *śāstras. Kīrtanam* is chanting about His glories, chanting the Hare Kṛṣṇa *mantra.* This is the beginning of the *bhakti-yoga* process. *Śravaṇam kīrtanaṁ viṣṇoḥ.* Everything is Viṣṇu, and meditation is on Viṣṇu. It is not possible to have *bhakti* without Viṣṇu. And Kṛṣṇa is the original form of Viṣṇu (*kṛṣṇas tu bhagavān svayam*). If we but follow this *bhakti-yoga* process, we shall be able to understand the Supreme, and all doubts will be removed.

The *aṣṭāṅga-yoga* process is outlined very specifically in the Sixth Chapter of the *Bhagavad-gītā* (6.13–14):

samaṁ kāya-śiro-grīvaṁ-dhārayann acalaṁ sthiraḥ
samprekṣya nāsikāgraṁ svaṁ diśaś cānavalokayan

praśāntātmā vigata-bhīr brahmacāri-vrate sthitaḥ
manaḥ saṁyamya mac-citto yukta āsīta mat-paraḥ

"One should hold one's body, neck, and head erect in a straight line and stare steadily at the tip of the nose. Thus, with an unagitated, subdued mind, devoid of fear, completely free from sex life, one should meditate upon Me within the heart and make Me the ultimate goal of life." *Yoga* does not mean going to a class, paying some money, performing some gymnastics, and then returning home to drink, smoke, and engage in sex. Such *yoga* is practiced by societies of the cheaters and the cheated. The authoritative *yoga* system is here outlined by the supreme authority, Śrī Kṛṣṇa Himself. Is there a better *yogī* than Kṛṣṇa, the Supreme Personality of Godhead? First of all, one has to go alone to a holy place and sit in a straight line, holding one's body, neck, and head erect, and stare steadily at the tip of the nose. Why is this? This is a method to help concentrate one's mind. That's all. The real purpose of *yoga*, however, is to remain always aware of Lord Kṛṣṇa within oneself.

One of the dangers of sitting in meditation is that one will fall asleep. I have seen many so-called meditators sitting and snoring. As soon as one closes his eyes, it is natural to feel sleepy; therefore it is recommended that one keep the eyes half closed and look at the tip of the nose. With one's sight thus concentrated, the mind should be subdued and unagitated. In India, the *yogī* often goes to a jungle to practice such meditation in solitude. But in a jungle, the *yogī* may think, "Maybe some tiger or snake is coming. What is that noise?" In this way, his mind may be agitated; therefore it is especially stated that the *yogī* must be "devoid of fear." A deerskin is especially recommended as a *yoga-āsana* because it contains a chemical property that repels snakes; thus the *yogī* will not be disturbed by serpents. Whatever the danger—serpents, tigers, or lions—

one can be truly fearless only when he is established in Kṛṣṇa consciousness. Due to perverted memory, the conditioned soul is naturally fearful. According to *Śrīmad-Bhāgavatam* (11.2.37), fear is due to forgetting one's eternal relationship with Kṛṣṇa (*bhayaṁ dvitīyābhiniveśataḥ syād īśād apetasya viparyayo 'smṛtiḥ*). Kṛṣṇa consciousness provides the only true basis for fearlessness; therefore perfect practice of *yoga* is not possible for one who is not Kṛṣṇa conscious.

The *yogī* must also be "completely free from sex life." If one indulges in sex, he cannot concentrate; therefore *brahmacarya*, complete celibacy, is recommended to make the mind steady. By practicing celibacy, one cultivates determination. One modern example of such determination is that of Mahatma Gandhi, who was determined to resist the powerful British empire by means of nonviolence. At this time India was dependent on the British, and the people had no weapons. The Britishers, being more powerful, easily cut down whatever violent revolutions the people attempted. Therefore Gandhi resorted to nonviolent noncooperation. "I shall not fight with the Britishers," he declared, "and even if they react with violence, I shall remain nonviolent. In this way the world will sympathize with us." Such a policy required a great amount of determination, and Gandhi's determination was very strong because he was a *brahmacārī*. Although he had children and a wife, he renounced sex at the age of thirty-six. It was this sexual renunciation that enabled him to be so determined that he was able to lead his country and drive the British from India.

Thus, refraining from sex enables one to be very determined and powerful. Even if you don't do anything else, just refraining from sex will make you very powerful. People do no know this secret. If you want to do something with determination, you have to refrain from sex. Regardless of the process—be it *haṭha-yoga*, *bhakti-yoga*, *jñāna-yoga*, or whatever—sex indulgence is not allowed. Sex is allowed only for householders who want to beget good children and raise them in Kṛṣṇa consciousness. Sex is not meant for sense enjoyment, although enjoyment is there by nature. Unless there is some enjoyment, why should one assume the responsibility of begetting children? That is the secret of nature's gift, but we should not take advantage of it. These are the secrets of life. By taking advantage and indulging in sex life, we are simply wasting our time. If one tells you that you can indulge in sex as much as you like and at the same time become a *yogī*, he is cheating you. If some so-called *guru* tells you to give him money in exchange for some *mantra* and that you can go on engaging in all kinds of nonsense, he is just cheating you. Because we want something sublime and yet want it cheaply, we put ourselves in a position to be cheated. This means that we actually want to be cheated. If we want something valuable, we must pay for it. We cannot expect to walk into a jewelry store and demand the most valuable jewel for a mere ten cents. No, we must pay a great deal. Similarly, if we want perfection in *yoga*, we have to pay by abstaining from sex. Perfection in *yoga* is not something childish, and the *Bhagavad-gītā* instructs us that if we try to make *yoga* into something childish, we will be cheated. There are many cheaters waiting to take our money, give us nothing, and leave. But according to Śrī Kṛṣṇa's authoritative statement in the *Bhagavad-gītā*, one must be "completely free from sex life." Being free from sex, one should "meditate upon Me within the heart and make Me the ultimate goal of life." This is real meditation.

Kṛṣṇa does not recommend meditation on the void. He specifically states, "Meditate upon Me." The *viṣṇu-mūrti* is situated in one's heart, and meditation upon Him is the object of *yoga*. This is the *sāṅkhya-yoga* system, as first practiced by Lord Kapiladeva, an incarnation of God. By sitting straight, staring steadily at the tip of one's nose, subduing one's mind, and abstaining from sex, one may be able to concentrate the mind on the *viṣṇu-mūrti* situated within the heart. When we refer to the Viṣṇu form, or *viṣṇu-mūrti*, we refer to Śrī Kṛṣṇa.

In the Kṛṣṇa consciousness movement we are meditating directly on Śrī Kṛṣṇa. This is a process of practical meditation. The members of this movement are concentrating their minds on Kṛṣṇa, regardless of their particular occupation. Someone may be working in the garden and digging in the earth, but he is thinking, "I am cultivating beautiful roses to offer to Kṛṣṇa." Someone else may be cooking in the kitchen, but he is always thinking, "I am preparing palatable food to be offered to Kṛṣṇa." Similarly, chanting and dancing in the temple are forms of meditating on Kṛṣṇa. Thus the boys and girls in this Society for Kṛṣṇa consciousness are perfect *yogīs* because they are meditating on Kṛṣṇa twenty-four hours a day. We are teaching the perfect *yoga* system, not according to our personal whims but according to the authority of the *Bhagavad-gītā.* Nothing is concocted or manufactured. The verses of the *Bhagavad-gītā* are there for all to see. The activities of the *bhakti-yogīs* in this movement are so molded that the practitioners cannot help but think of Kṛṣṇa at all times. "Meditate upon Me within the heart, and make Me the ultimate goal of life," Śrī Kṛṣṇa says. This is the perfect *yoga* system, and one who practices it prepares himself to be transferred to Kṛṣṇaloka.

yuñjann evaṁ sadātmānaṁ yogī niyata-mānasaḥ
śāntiṁ nirvāṇa-paramāṁ mat-saṁsthām adhigacchati

"Thus practicing constant control of the body, mind, and activities, the mystic transcendentalist, his mind regulated, attains to the kingdom of God [or the abode of Kṛṣṇa] by cessation of material existence." (Bg. 6.15)

It is stated in Sanskrit in this verse, *śāntiṁ nirvāṇa-paramām;* that is, one attains peace through *nirvāṇa-paramām,* or the cessation of material activities. *Nirvāṇa* refers not to the void but to putting an end to materialistic activities. Unless one puts an end to them, there is no question of peace. When Hiraṇyakaśipu asked his five-year-old son Prahlāda Mahārāja, "My dear boy, what is the best thing you have learned thus far?" Prahlāda immediately replied, *tat sādhu manye 'sura-varya dehināṁ sadā samudvigna-dhiyām asad-grahāt:* "My dear father, O greatest of the demons, materialistic people are always full of anxiety because they have accepted as real that which is impermanent." The word *asad-grahāt* is important because it indicates that materialists are always hankering to capture or possess something that is impermanent. History affords us many examples. Mr. John Kennedy was a very rich man who wanted to become President, and he spent a great deal of money to attain that elevated position. Yet although he had a nice wife, children, and the presidency, everything was finished within a second. In the material world people are always trying to capture something that is impermanent. Unfortunately, people do not come to their senses and realize, "I am permanent. I am spirit soul. Why am I hankering after something that is impermanent?"

We are always busy acquiring comforts for the body without considering that today, tomorrow, or in a hundred years the body will be finished. As far as the real "I" is concerned, "I am spirit soul. I have no birth. I have no death. What, then, is my proper function?" When we act on the material platform we are engaged in bodily functions; therefore Prahlāda Mahārāja says that people are anxious because all their activities are targeted to capturing and possessing something impermanent. All living entities—men, beasts, birds, or whatever—are always full of anxiety, and this is the material disease. If we are always full of anxiety, how can we attain peace? People may live in a very nice house, but out front they place signs saying "Beware of Dog" or "No Trespassers." This means that although they are living comfortably, they are anxious that someone will come and molest them. A man sitting in an office and earning a very good salary is always thinking, "Oh, I hope I don't lose this position." The American nation is very rich, but because of this it has to maintain a great defense force. So who is free from anxiety? The conclusion is that if we want peace without anxiety, we have to come to Kṛṣṇa consciousness. There is no alternative.

In order to attain peace, we must meditate on Kṛṣṇa, and by meditating on Kṛṣṇa we can control the body. The first part of the body to control is the tongue, and the next part is the genital. When these are controlled, everything is controlled. The tongue is controlled by chanting Hare Kṛṣṇa and by eating *kṛṣṇa-prasādam.* As soon as the tongue is controlled, the stomach is controlled, and next the genitals are controlled. Actually, controlling the body and mind is a very simple process. When the mind is fixed on Kṛṣṇa and has no other engagement, it is automatically controlled. Activities should always be centered on working for Kṛṣṇa—gardening, typing, cooking, cleaning, whatever. By engaging the body, mind, and activities in the service of Kṛṣṇa, one attains the supreme *nirvāṇa,* which abides in Kṛṣṇa. Everything is in Kṛṣṇa; therefore we cannot find peace outside Kṛṣṇa conscious activities.

The ultimate goal of *yoga* is thus clearly explained. *Yoga* is not meant for attaining any kind of material facility; it is to enable the cessation of all material existence. As long as we require some material facilities, we will get them. But these facilities will not solve the problems of life. I have traveled throughout the world, and it is my opinion that American boys and girls have the best material facilities. But does this mean they have attained peace? Can anyone say, "Yes, I am completely peaceful"? If this is so, why are American youngsters so frustrated and confused?

As long as we practice *yoga* in order to attain some material facility, there will be no question of peace. *Yoga* should only be practiced in order to understand Kṛṣṇa. *Yoga* is meant for the reestablishment of our lost relationship with Kṛṣṇa. Generally, one joins a *yoga* society in order to improve health, often to reduce fat. People in rich nations eat more than necessary, become fat, and then pay exorbitant prices to so-called *yoga* instructors in order to reduce. People try to reduce their weight by all these artificial gymnastics; they do not understand that if they just eat vegetables and grains and light foods, they will never get fat. People get fat because they eat voraciously. Those who eat voraciously suffer from diabetes, overweight, heart attacks, etc., and those who eat insufficiently suffer from such diseases as tuberculosis. Therefore moderation is required, and moderation in eating means that we eat only what is needed to keep body and soul together. If we eat more than we need or less, we will become diseased. All this is explained in the following verses:

nāty-aśnatas tu yogo 'sti na caikāntam anaśnataḥ
na cāti-svapna-śīlasya jāgrato naiva cārjuna

"There is no possibility of one's becoming a *yogī*, O Arjuna, if one eats too much or eats too little, sleeps too much or does not sleep enough." (Bg. 6.16)

yuktāhāra-vihārasya yukta-ceṣṭasya karmasu
yukta-svapnāvabodhasya yogo bhavati duḥkha-hā

"He who is regulated in his habits of eating, sleeping, recreation, and work can mitigate all material pains by practicing *yoga*." (Bg. 6.17) It is not that we are to starve ourselves. The body must be kept fit for any practice; therefore eating is required, and according to our program, we eat only *kṛṣṇa-prasādam.* If you can comfortably eat ten pounds of food a day, then eat it, but if you try to eat ten pounds out of greed or avarice, you will suffer.

So in the practice of Kṛṣṇa consciousness, all these activities are present, but they are spiritualized. The cessation of material existence does not mean entering into "the void," which is only a myth. There is no void anywhere within the creation of the Lord. I am not void but spirit soul. If I were void, how could my bodily development take place? Where is this "void"? If we sow a seed in the ground, it grows into a plant or large tree. Similarly, the father injects a seed into the womb of the mother, and the body grows like a tree. Where is the void? In the Fourteenth Chapter of the *Bhagavad-gītā* (14.4), Śrī Kṛṣṇa states,

sarva-yoniṣu kaunteya mūrtayaḥ sambhavanti yāḥ
tāsāṁ brahma mahad yonir ahaṁ bīja-pradaḥ pitā

"It should be understood that all species of life, O son of Kuntī, are made possible by birth in this material nature, and that I am the seed-giving father." Originally Kṛṣṇa gives the seed by placing it in the womb of material nature, and thus many living entities are generated. How can one argue against this process? If the seed of existence is void, how has this body developed?

Nirvāṇa actually means not accepting another material body. It's not that we attempt to make this body void. *Nirvāṇa* means making the miserable, material, conditioned body void—that is, converting the material body into a spiritual body. This means entering into the kingdom of God, which is described in the Fifteenth Chapter of the *Bhagavad-gītā* (15.6):

na tad bhāsayate sūryo sa śaśāṅko na pāvakaḥ
yad gatvā na nivartante tad dhāma paramaṁ mama

"That abode of Mine is not illumined by the sun or moon, nor by fire or electricity. Those who reach it never return to this material world."

So there is no void anywhere within the Lord's creation. All the planets in the spiritual sky are self-illumined, like the sun. The kingdom of God is everywhere, but the spiritual sky and the planets thereof are all *paraṁ dhāma,* or superior abodes. As stated, neither sunlight, moonlight, nor electricity are required in the *paraṁ dhāma.* We cannot find such an abode within this universe. We may travel as far as possible in our spaceships, but we will not find anyplace where there is no sunlight. The sunlight is so extensive that it pervades the universe. Therefore, that abode in which there is no sunlight, moonlight, or electricity must be beyond the material sky. Beyond the material nature is the spiritual nature. Actually, we know practically nothing of the material nature; we do not even know how it was originally formed. So how can we know anything about the spiritual nature beyond? We have to learn from Kṛṣṇa, who lives there; otherwise we will remain in ignorance.

In the *Bhagavad-gītā,* information of the spiritual sky is given. How can we know anything about that which we cannot reach? Our senses are so imperfect, how can we attain such knowledge? We just have to hear from the right source and accept. How can we ever know who our father is unless we accept the word of our mother? Our mother says, "Here is your father," and we have to accept this. We cannot determine the identity of our father by making inquiries here and there or by experimenting. This knowledge is beyond our means. Similarly, if we want to learn about the spiritual sky, God's kingdom, we have to hear from the authority, mother *Vedas.* The *Vedas* are called *veda-mātā,* or mother *Vedas,* because the knowledge imparted therein is like that knowledge received from the mother. We *have* to believe in order to acquire knowledge. There is no possibility of acquiring this transcendental knowledge by experimenting with our imperfect senses.

In the *Bhagavad-gītā* (6.15) Lord Kṛṣṇa states, *śāntiṁ nirvāṇa-paramāṁ mat-saṁsthām adhigacchati.* This means that a consummate *yogī,* who is perfect in understanding Lord Kṛṣṇa, can attain real peace and ultimately reach the supreme abode of the Lord. This abode is known as Kṛṣṇaloka, or Goloka Vṛndāvana. In the *Brahma-saṁhitā* it is clearly stated that the Lord, although residing always in His abode called Goloka, is the all-pervading Brahman and the localized Paramātmā as well by dint of His superior spiritual energies (*goloka eva nivasaty akhilātma-bhūtaḥ*). He is like the sun, which is millions of miles away and yet is still present within this room by dint of its rays. No one can reach the spiritual sky or enter into the eternal abode of the Lord (either Vaikuṇṭha or Goloka Vṛndāvana) without properly understanding Kṛṣṇa and His plenary expansion Viṣṇu. And according to the *Brahma-saṁhitā*, it is necessary to learn this knowledge from our authorized mother (*veda-mātā*), the Vedic literature.

In conclusion, the person who works in Kṛṣṇa consciousness is the perfect *yogī* because his mind is always absorbed in Kṛṣṇa's activities. *Sa vai manaḥ kṛṣṇa-padāravindayoḥ.* In the *Vedas* we also learn, *tam eva viditvāti mṛtyum eti:* "One can overcome the path of birth and death only by understanding the Supreme Personality of Godhead, Kṛṣṇa." Thus perfection of *yoga* is the attainment of freedom from material existence and not some magical jugglery or gymnastic feats meant to befool innocent people.

In this system of *yoga*, moderation is required; therefore it is stated that we should not eat too much or too little, sleep too much or too little, or work too much or too little. All these activities are there because we have to execute the *yoga* system with the material body. In other words, we have to make the best use of a bad bargain. The material body is a bad bargain because it is the source of all miseries. In our normal, healthy condition as pure spirit soul, we do not experience any misery. Misery and disease occur due to material contamination or infection. So material existence is a diseased condition of the soul. And what is that disease? The disease is this body. This body is actually not meant for me. It may be "my" body, but it is a symptom of my diseased condition. In any case, I should identify with this body no more than I would identify with my clothes. In this world, we are all differently dressed. We are dressed as red men, brown men, white men, black men, yellow men, etc., or as Indians, Americans, Hindus, Muslims, Christians, etc. All these designations are not symptomatic of our actual position but of our diseased condition. The *yoga* system is meant to cure this disease by connecting us again with the Supreme Lord.

We are meant to be connected with the Supreme Lord just as our hand is meant to be connected to our body. We are part and parcel of the Supreme Lord, just as the hand is part and parcel of the body. When the hand is severed from the body, it is valueless, but when it is joined to the body, it is invaluable. Similarly, in our material condition we are disconnected from God. Actually, the word *disconnected* is not precise, because the connection is always there. God is always supplying all our necessities. Since nothing can exist without Kṛṣṇa, we cannot be disconnected from Him. Rather, it is better to say that we have forgotten that we are connected to Kṛṣṇa. Because of this forgetfulness, we have entered the criminal department of the universe. The government still takes care of its criminals, but they are legally disconnected from the civilian state. Our disconnection is a result of our engaging in so many nonsensical activities instead of utilizing our senses in the performance of our Kṛṣṇa conscious duties.

Instead of thinking "I am the eternal servant of God, or Kṛṣṇa," we are thinking "I am the servant of my society, my country, my husband, my wife, my dog . . ." This is called forgetfulness. How has this come about? All these misconceptions have arisen due to this body. Because I was born in America, I am thinking that I am an American. Each society teaches its citizens to think in this way. Because I am thinking that I am an American, the American government can tell me, "Come and fight. Give your life for your country." This is all due to the bodily conception; therefore an intelligent person should know that he is suffering miseries due to his body and that he should not act in such a way that he will continue to be imprisoned within a material body birth after birth. According to *Padma Purāṇa*, there are 8,400,000 species of life, and all are but different forms of contamination—whether one has an American body, an Indian body, a dog's body, a hog's body, or whatever. Therefore the first instruction in *yoga* is "I am not this body."

Attaining liberation from the contamination of the material body is the first teaching of the *Bhagavad-gītā*. In the Second Chapter, after Arjuna told Śrī Kṛṣṇa "I shall not fight," the Lord said, "While speaking learned words, you are mourning for what is not worthy of grief. Those who are wise lament for neither the living nor the dead." (Bg. 2.11) In other words, Arjuna was thinking on the bodily platform. He wanted to leave the battlefield because he did not want to fight with his relatives. All his conceptions were within the bodily atmosphere; therefore after Arjuna accepted Śrī Kṛṣṇa as his spiritual master, the Lord immediately chastised him in order to teach him. Essentially, Śrī Kṛṣṇa told Arjuna, "You are talking very wisely, as if you know so many things, but actually you are speaking nonsense because you are speaking from the bodily position." Similarly, people throughout the world are posing themselves as highly advanced in education, science, philosophy, politics, etc., but their position is on the bodily platform.

A vulture may rise very high in the sky—thousands of feet—and it is wonderful to see him fly in this way. He also has powerful eyes, for he can spot a carcass from a great distance. Yet what is the object of all these great qualifications? A dead body, a rotting carcass. His perfection is just to discover a dead piece of meat and eat it. That's all. Similarly, we may have a very high education, but what is our objective? Sense enjoyment, the enjoyment of this material body. We may rise very high with our spaceships, but what is the purpose? Sense gratification, that's all. This means that all the striving and all this high education are merely on the animal platform.

Therefore we should first of all know that our miserable material condition is due to this body. At the same time, we should know that this body is not permanent. Although I identify with my body, family, society, country, and so many other things, how long will these objects exist? They are not permanent. *Asat* is a word meaning that they will cease to exist. *Asann api kleśada āsa dehaḥ.:* "The body is simply troublesome and impermanent."

Many people come to us saying, "Swāmījī, my position is so troublesome," but as soon as we suggest the medicine, they will not accept it. This means that people want to manufacture their own medicine. Why do we go to a physician if we want to treat ourselves? People want to accept only what they think is palatable.

Although we are suggesting that this body is a form of contamination, we are not recommending that it be abused. We may use a car to carry us to work, but this does not mean that we should not take care of the car. We should take care of the car for it to carry us to and fro, but we should not become so attached to it that we are polishing it every day. We must utilize the material body in order to execute Kṛṣṇa consciousness, and to this end we should keep it fit and healthy, but we should not become too attached to it. That is called *yukta-vairāgya.* The body should not be neglected. We should bathe regularly, eat regularly, and sleep regularly in order to keep mind and body healthy. Some people say that the body should be renounced and that we should take some drugs and abandon ourselves to intoxication, but this is not a *yoga* process. Kṛṣṇa has given us nice food—fruits, grains, vegetables, and milk—and we can prepare hundreds and thousands of nice preparations and offer them to the Lord. Our process is to eat *kṛṣṇa-prasādam* and to satisfy the tongue in that way. But we should not be greedy and eat dozens of *samosās,* sweetballs, and *rasagullās.* No. We should eat and sleep just enough to keep the body fit, and no more. It is stated,

yuktāhāra-vihārasya yukta-ceṣṭasya karmasu
yukta-svapnāvabodhasya yogo bhavati duḥkha-hā

"He who is temperate in his habits of eating, sleeping, recreation, and work can mitigate all material pains by practicing the *yoga* system." (Bg. 6.17)

Although we should minimize our eating and sleeping, we should not attempt this too rapidly, at the risk of becoming sick. Because people are accustomed to eating voraciously, there are prescriptions for fasting. We can reduce our sleeping and eating, but we should remain in good health for spiritual purposes. We should not attempt to reduce eating and sleeping too rapidly or artificially; when we advance we will naturally not feel pain due to the reduction of these natural bodily processes. In this respect, Raghunātha dāsa Gosvāmī offers a good example. Although a very rich man's son, Raghunātha dāsa left his home to join Lord Caitanya Mahāprabhu. Because he was the only son, Raghunātha dāsa was very beloved by his father. Understanding that his son had gone to Jagannātha Purī to join Lord Caitanya, the father sent four servants with money to attend him. At first Raghunātha accepted the money, thinking, "Oh, since my father has sent all this money, I will accept it and regularly invite all the *sannyāsīs* to a feast."

After some time, however, the feasts came to an end. Lord Caitanya Mahāprabhu then inquired from His secretary, Svarūpa Dāmodara, "Nowadays I don't receive any invitations from Raghunātha. What has happened?"

"That is because Raghunātha has stopped accepting his father's money."

"Oh, that's very nice," Caitanya Mahāprabhu said.

"Raghunātha was thinking, 'Although I have renounced everything, I am still enjoying my father's money. This is hypocritical.' Therefore he has told the servants to go home and has refused the money."

"So how is he living?" Caitanya Mahāprabhu inquired.

"Oh, he's standing on the steps of the Jagannātha temple, and when the priests pass him on their way home, they offer him some *prasādam*. In this way, he is satisfied."

"This is very nice," Caitanya Mahāprabhu commented.

Regularly going to the Jagannātha temple, Lord Caitanya Mahāprabhu would see Raghunātha standing on the steps. After a few days, however, He no longer saw him there. Therefore the Lord commented to His secretary, "I no longer see Raghunātha standing on the temple steps."

"He has given that up," Svarūpa Dāmodara explained. "He was thinking, 'Oh, I am standing here just like a prostitute, waiting for someone to come and give me food. No. I don't like this at all.'"

"That is very nice," Caitanya Mahāprabhu said, "but how is he eating?"

"Every day he is collecting some rejected rice from the kitchen and is eating that."

To encourage Raghunātha, Caitanya Mahāprabhu one day visited him. "Raghunātha," the Lord said, "I hear that you are eating very palatable food. Why are you not inviting Me?"

Raghunātha did not reply, but the Lord quickly found the place where he kept the rice, and then the Lord immediately took some and began to eat it.

"Dear Lord," Raghunātha implored, "please do not eat this. It is not fit for You."

"Oh, no? Why are you saying it is not fit for Me? It is

Lord Jagannātha's *prasādam*!"

Lord Caitanya Mahāprabhu enacted this pastime just to discourage Raghunātha from thinking "I am eating this miserable, rejected rice." Through the Lord's encouragement, Raghunātha dāsa Gosvāmī reduced his daily quantity of food until he was finally eating only one pat of butter every other day. And every day he was also bowing down hundreds of times and constantly chanting the holy names. *Saṅkhyā-pūrvaka-nāma-gāna-natibhiḥ kālāvasānī-kṛtau.*

Although this is an excellent example of minimizing all material necessities, we should not try to imitate it. It is not possible for an ordinary man to imitate Raghunātha dāsa Gosvāmī, who was one of the six Gosvāmīs, a highly elevated associate of Lord Caitanya Mahāprabhu Himself. Each one of the six Gosvāmīs displayed a unique example of how one can advance in Kṛṣṇa consciousness, but it is not our duty to imitate them. We should just try to follow, as far as possible, in their footsteps. If we immediately try to become like Raghunātha dāsa Gosvāmī by imitating him, we are sure to fail, and whatever progress we have made will be destroyed. Therefore the Lord says (Bg. 6.16) that there is no possibility of one's becoming a *yogī* if one eats too much or too little.

The same moderation applies to sleep. Presently I may be sleeping ten hours a day, but if I can keep myself fit by sleeping five hours, why sleep ten? As far as the body is concerned, there are four demands—eating, sleeping, mating, and defending. The problem with modern civilization is that it is trying to increase these demands, but they should be decreased instead. Eat what we need and sleep when we need, and our health will be excellent. There is no question of artificial imitation.

And what is the result obtained by one who is temperate in his habits?

yadā viniyataṁ cittam ātmany evāvatiṣṭhate
nispṛhaḥ sarva-kāmebhyo yukta ity ucyate tadā

"When the *yogī*, by practice of *yoga*, disciplines his mental activities and becomes situated in transcendence—devoid of all material desires—he is said to have attained *yoga*." (Bg. 6.18)

The perfection of *yoga* means keeping the mind in a state of equilibrium. Materially speaking, this is impossible. After reading a mundane novel once, you will not want to read it again, but you can read the *Bhagavad-gītā* four times a day and still not tire of it. You may chant some ordinary person's name a half an hour, or sing a mundane song three or four times, but before long this becomes tiresome. The Hare Kṛṣṇa *mantra,* however, can be chanted day and night and one will never tire of it. Therefore it is only through transcendental vibration that the mind can be kept in a state of equilibrium. When one's mental activities are thus stabilized, one is said to have attained *yoga.*

The perfectional stage of *yoga* was exhibited by King Ambarīṣa, who utilized all his senses in the service of the Lord. As stated in *Śrīmad-Bhāgavatam* (9.4.18–20),

sa vai manaḥ kṛṣṇa-padāravindayor
vacāṁsi vaikuṇṭha-guṇānuvarṇane
karau harer mandira-mārjanādiṣu
śrutiṁ cakārācyuta-sat-kathodaye

mukunda-liṅgālaya-darśane dṛśau
tad-bhṛtya-gātra-sparśe 'ṅga-saṅgamam
ghrāṇaṁ ca tat-pāda-saroja-saurabhe
śrīmat-tulasyā rasanaṁ tad-arpite

pādau hareḥ kṣetra-padānusarpaṇe
śiro hṛṣīkeśa-padābhivandane
kāmaṁ ca dāsye na tu kāma-kāmyayā
yathottamaśloka-janāśrayā ratiḥ

"King Ambarīṣa first of all engaged his mind on the lotus feet of Lord Kṛṣṇa; then, one after another, he engaged his words in describing the transcendental qualities of the Lord, his hands in mopping the temple of the Lord, his ears in hearing of the activities of the Lord, his eyes in seeing the transcendental forms of the Lord, his body in touching the bodies of the devotees, his sense of smell in smelling the scents of the lotus flowers offered to the Lord, his tongue in tasting the *tulasī* leaves offered at the temple of the Lord, his head in offering obeisances unto the Lord, and his desires in executing the mission of the Lord. All these transcendental activities are quite befitting a pure devotee."

This, then, is the perfection of *yoga*—to be devoid of all material desire. If all our desires are for Kṛṣṇa, there is no scope for material desire. All material desire is automatically finished. We don't have to try to concentrate artificially. All perfection is there in Kṛṣṇa consciousness because it is on the spiritual platform. Being on the spiritual platform, this supreme *yoga* is eternal, blissful, and full of knowledge. Therefore there are no misgivings or material impediments.

5

Determination and Steadiness in Yoga

yathā dīpo nivāta-stho neṅgate sopamā smṛtā
yogino yata-cittasya yuñjato yogam ātmanaḥ

"As a lamp in a windless place does not waver, so the transcendentalist whose mind is controlled remains always steady in his meditation on the transcendent Self." (Bg. 6.19)

If the mind is absorbed in Kṛṣṇa consciousness, it will remain as steady as the flame of a candle that is in a room where there is no wind. Therefore it is said that a truly Kṛṣṇa conscious person always absorbed in transcendence, in constant undisturbed meditation on his worshipable Lord, is as steady as a lamp or candle in a windless place. Just as the flame is not agitated, the mind is not agitated, and that steadiness is the perfection of *yoga.*

The state of one thus steadily situated in meditation on the transcendent Self, or the Supreme Lord, is described by Śrī Kṛṣṇa in the following verses of the *Bhagavad-gītā* (6.20–23):

yatroparamate cittaṁ niruddhaṁ yoga-sevayā
yatra caivātmanātmānaṁ paśyann ātmani tuṣyati

sukham ātyantikaṁ yat tad buddhi-grāhyam atīndriyam
vetti yatra na caivāyaṁ sthitaś calati tattvataḥ

yaṁ labdhvā cāparaṁ lābhaṁ manyate nādhikaṁ tataḥ
yasmin sthito na duḥkhena guruṇāpi vicālyate

taṁ vidyād duḥkha-saṁyoga-viyogaṁ yoga-saṁjñitam

"In the stage of perfection called trance, or *samādhi,* one's mind is completely restrained from material mental activities by the practice of *yoga.* This perfection is characterized by one's ability to see the Self by the pure mind and to relish and rejoice in the Self. In that joyous state one is situated in boundless transcendental happiness, realized through transcendental senses. Established thus, one never departs from the truth, and upon gaining this he thinks there is no greater gain. Being situated in such a position, one is never shaken, even in the midst of the greatest difficulty. This indeed is actual freedom from all miseries arising from material contact."

Samādhi does not mean making oneself void or merging into the void. That is impossible. *Kleśo 'dhikataras teṣām avyaktāsakta-cetasām.* Some *yogīs* say that one has to put an end to all activities and make oneself motionless. But how is this possible? By nature the living entity is a moving, acting spirit. "Motionless" means putting an end to material motion and being fixed in Kṛṣṇa consciousness. In such a state, one is no longer disturbed by material propensities. As one becomes materially motionless, one's motions in Kṛṣṇa consciousness increase. As one becomes active in Kṛṣṇa consciousness, one becomes automatically motionless in respect to material activities.

I have often used the example of a restless child. Since it is impossible to make such a child motionless, it is necessary to give him some playthings or some pictures to look at. In this way he will be motionless in the sense that he will not be committing some mischief. But if one really wants to make him motionless, one must give him some engagement in Kṛṣṇa consciousness. Then there will be no scope for mischievous activities, due to realization in Kṛṣṇa consciousness. To be engaged in Kṛṣṇa consciousness one should first realize, "I am Kṛṣṇa's. I do not belong to matter. I do not belong to this nation or that society. I do not belong to this rascal or that rascal. I am simply Kṛṣṇa's." This is full knowledge—realization of our actual position as part and parcel of Kṛṣṇa. As Kṛṣṇa states in the Fifteenth Chapter (Bg. 15.7), *mamaivāṁśo jīva-loke:* "The living entities in this conditioned world are My eternal fragmental parts." As soon as we understand this, we immediately cease our material activities, and this is what is meant by being motionless. In this state, one sees the Self by the pure mind and relishes and rejoices in the Self. "Pure mind" means understanding "I belong to Kṛṣṇa." At the present moment the mind is contaminated because we are thinking "I belong to this, I belong to that." The mind is pure when it understands, "I belong to Kṛṣṇa."

Rejoicing in the Self means rejoicing with Kṛṣṇa. Kṛṣṇa is the Supersoul, or the Superself. I am the individual soul, or the individual self. The Superself and the self enjoy together. Enjoyment cannot be alone; there must be two. What experience do we have of solitary enjoyment? Solitary enjoyment is not possible. Enjoyment means two: Kṛṣṇa, who is the Supersoul, and the individual soul.

If one is convinced that "I am part and parcel of Kṛṣṇa," one is not disturbed even in the midst of the greatest difficulties, because one knows that Kṛṣṇa will give protection. That is surrender. To attain this position one must try his best, use his intelligence, and believe in Kṛṣṇa. *Bālasya neha śaraṇaṁ pitarau nṛsiṁha* (*Bhāg.* 7.9.19). If Kṛṣṇa does not protect us, nothing can save us. If Kṛṣṇa neglects us, there is no remedy, and whatever measures we take to try to protect ourselves will ultimately be defeated. There may be many expert physicians treating a diseased man, but that is no guarantee he will live. If Kṛṣṇa so wills, a person will die despite the best physicians and medicines. On the other hand, if Kṛṣṇa is protecting us, we will survive even without medical treatment. When one is fully surrendered to Kṛṣṇa, he becomes happy, knowing that regardless of the situation, Kṛṣṇa will protect him. He is just like a child who is fully surrendered to his parents, confident that they are there to protect him. As stated by Yāmunācārya in his *Stotra-ratna* (43), *kadāham aikāntika-nitya-kiṅkaraḥ praharṣayiṣyāmi sanātha jīvitam:* "O Lord, when shall I engage as Your permanent, eternal servant and always feel joyful to have such a perfect master?" If we know that there is someone very powerful who is our patron and savior, aren't we happy? But if we try to act on our own and at our own risk, how can we be happy? Happiness means being in Kṛṣṇa consciousness and being convinced that "Kṛṣṇa will give me protection," and being true to Kṛṣṇa. It is not possible to be happy otherwise.

Of course, Kṛṣṇa is giving all living entities protection, even in their rebellious condition (*eko bahūnāṁ yo vidadhāti kāmān*). Without Kṛṣṇa's protection, we cannot live for a second. When we admit and recognize Kṛṣṇa's kindness, we become happy. Kṛṣṇa is protecting us at every moment, but we fail to realize this because we have taken life at our own risk. Kṛṣṇa gives us a certain amount of freedom, saying, "All right, do whatever you like. As far as possible, I will give you protection." However, when the living entity is fully surrendered to Kṛṣṇa, Kṛṣṇa takes total charge and gives special protection. If a child grows up and doesn't care for his father and acts freely, what can his father do? He can only say, "Do whatever you like." But when a son puts himself fully under his father's protection, he receives more care. As Kṛṣṇa states in the Ninth Chapter of the *Bhagavad-gītā* (9.29),

samo 'haṁ sarva-bhūteṣu na me dveṣyo 'sti na priyaḥ
ye bhajanti tu māṁ bhaktyā mayi te teṣu cāpy aham

"I envy no one, nor am I partial to anyone. I am equal to all. But whoever renders service unto Me in devotion is a friend—is in Me—and I am also a friend to him."

How can Kṛṣṇa be envious of anyone? Everyone is Kṛṣṇa's son. Similarly, how can Kṛṣṇa be an enemy toward anyone? Since all living entities are Kṛṣṇa's sons, He is everyone's friend. Unfortunately, we are not taking advantage of His friendship, and that is our disease. Once we recognize Kṛṣṇa as our eternal father and friend, we can understand that He is always protecting us, and in this way we can be happy.

sa niścayena yoktavyo yogo 'nirviṇṇa-cetasā
saṅkalpa-prabhavān kāmāṁs tyaktvā sarvān aśeṣataḥ
manasaivendriya-grāmaṁ viniyamya samantataḥ

"One should engage oneself in the practice of *yoga* with determination and faith and not be deviated from the path. One should abandon, without exception, all material desires born of mental speculation and thus control all the senses on all sides by the mind." (Bg. 6.24)

As stated before, this determination can be attained only by one who does not indulge in sex. Celibacy makes one's determination strong; therefore, from the very beginning Kṛṣṇa states that the *yogī* does not engage in sex. If one indulges in sex, one's determination will be flickering. Therefore sex life should be controlled according to the rules and regulations governing the *gṛhastha-āśrama*, or sex should be given up altogether. Actually, it should be given up altogether, but if this is not possible, it should be controlled. Then determination will come because, after all, determination is a bodily affair. Determination means continuing to practice Kṛṣṇa consciousness with patience and perseverance. If one does not immediately attain the desired results, one should not think, "Oh, what is this Kṛṣṇa consciousness? I will give it up." No, we must have determination and faith in Kṛṣṇa's words.

In this regard there is a mundane example. When a young girl gets married, she immediately hankers for a child. She thinks, "Now I am married. I must have a child immediately." But how is this possible? The girl must have patience, become a faithful wife, serve her husband, and let her love grow. Eventually, because she is married, it is certain that she will have a child. Similarly, when we are in Kṛṣṇa consciousness, our perfection is guaranteed, but we must have patience and determination. We should think, "I must execute my duties and should not be impatient." Impatience is due to loss of determination, and loss of determination is due to excessive sex.

The *yogī* should be determined and should patiently prosecute Kṛṣṇa consciousness without deviation. One should be sure of success at the end and pursue this course with great perseverance, not becoming discouraged if there is any delay in the attainment of success. Success is sure for the rigid practitioner. Regarding *bhakti-yoga*, Rūpa Gosvāmī says,

utsāhān niścayād dhairyāt tat-tat-karma-pravartanāt
saṅga-tyāgāt sato vṛtteḥ ṣaḍbhir bhaktiḥ prasidhyati

"One can achieve success in *bhakti-yoga* by executing the process with full-hearted enthusiasm, perseverance, and determination, by following the prescribed duties, by rejecting the association of nondevotees, and by engaging completely in activities of goodness." (*Upadeśāmṛta* 3)

As for determination, one should follow the example of the sparrow who lost her eggs in the waves of the ocean. Once a sparrow laid her eggs on the shore of the ocean, but the big ocean carried away the eggs on its waves. The sparrow became very upset and asked the ocean to return her eggs. The ocean did not even consider her appeal. So the sparrow decided to dry up the ocean. She began to peck at the water with her small beak, and everyone laughed at her for her impossible determination. The news of her activity spread, and when at last Garuḍa, the gigantic bird carrier of Lord Viṣṇu, heard it, he became compassionate toward his small sister bird, and so he came to see her. Garuḍa was very pleased by the determination of the small sparrow, and he promised to help. Thus Garuḍa at once asked the ocean to return her eggs lest he himself take up the work of the sparrow. The ocean was frightened by this and returned the eggs. Thus the sparrow became happy by the grace of Garuḍa.

Similarly, the practice of *yoga*, especially *bhakti-yoga* in Kṛṣṇa consciousness, may appear to be a very difficult job. But if anyone follows the principles with great determination, the Lord will surely help, for God helps those who help themselves.

śanaiḥ śanair uparamed buddhyā dhṛti-gṛhītayā
ātma-saṁsthaṁ manaḥ kṛtvā na kiñcid api cintayet

"Gradually, step by step, one should become situated in trance by means of intelligence sustained by full conviction, and thus the mind should be fixed on the Self alone and should think of nothing else." (Bg. 6.25)

We are the self, and Kṛṣṇa is also the Self. When there is sunlight, we can see the sun and ourselves also. However, when there is dense darkness, we sometimes cannot even see our own body. Although the body is there, the darkness is so dense that I cannot see myself. But when the sunshine is present, I can see myself as well as the sun. Similarly, seeing the self means first of all seeing the Supreme Self, Kṛṣṇa. In the *Kaṭha Upaniṣad* it is stated, *nityo nityānāṁ cetanaś cetanānām:* "The Supreme Self is the chief eternal of all eternals, and He is the chief living being of all living beings." Kṛṣṇa consciousness means fixing the mind on Kṛṣṇa, and when the mind is thus fixed, it is fixed on the complete whole. If the stomach is cared for and supplied nutritious food, all the bodily limbs are nourished, and we are in good health. Similarly, if we water the root of a tree, all the branches, leaves, flowers, and twigs are automatically taken care of. By rendering service to Kṛṣṇa, we automatically render the best service to all others.

As stated before, a Kṛṣṇa conscious person does not sit down idly. He knows that Kṛṣṇa consciousness is such an important philosophy that it should be distributed. Therefore the members of the Kṛṣṇa consciousness society are not just sitting in the temple but are going out on *saṅkīrtana* parties, preaching and distributing this supreme philosophy. That is the mission of Śrī Kṛṣṇa Caitanya Mahāprabhu and His followers. Other *yogīs* may be satisfied with their own elevation and sit in secluded places practicing *yoga.* For them, *yoga* is nothing more than their personal concern. A devotee, however, is not satisfied just in elevating his personal self.

vāñchā-kalpatarubhyaś ca kṛpā-sindhubhya eva ca
patitānāṁ pāvanebhyo vaiṣṇavebhyo namo namaḥ

"I offer my respectful obeisances unto all the Vaiṣṇava devotees of the Lord, who can fulfill the desires of everyone, just like desire trees, and who are full of compassion for the fallen souls." A devotee displays great compassion toward conditioned souls. The word *kṛpā* means "mercy," and *sindhu* means "ocean." A devotee is an ocean of mercy, and he naturally wants to distribute this mercy. Lord Jesus Christ, for instance, was God conscious, Kṛṣṇa conscious, but he was not satisfied in keeping this knowledge within himself. Had he continued to live alone in God consciousness, he would not have met crucifixion. But no. Being a devotee and naturally compassionate, he also wanted to take care of others by making them God conscious. Although he was forbidden to preach God consciousness, he continued to do so at the risk of his own life. This is the nature of a devotee.

It is therefore stated in the *Bhagavad-gītā* (18.68–69) that the devotee who preaches is most dear to the Lord.

ya idaṁ paramaṁ guhyaṁ mad-bhakteṣv abhidhāsyati
bhaktiṁ mayi parāṁ kṛtvā mām evaiṣyaty asaṁśayaḥ

"For one who explains the supreme secret of the *Bhagavad-gītā* to the devotees, devotional service is guaranteed, and at the end he will come back to Me."

na ca tasmān manuṣyeṣu kaścin me priya-kṛttamaḥ
bhavitā na ca me tasmād anyaḥ priyataro bhuvi

"There is no servant in this world more dear to Me than he, nor will there ever be one more dear." Therefore the devotees go out to preach, and going forth, they sometimes meet opposing elements. Sometimes they are defeated, sometimes disappointed, sometimes able to convince, sometimes unable. It is not that every devotee is well equipped to preach. Just as there are different types of people, there are three classes of devotees. In the third class are those who have no faith. If they are engaged in devotional service officially, for some ulterior purpose, they cannot achieve the highest perfectional stage. Most probably they will slip after some time. At present they may be engaged in devotional service, but because they do not develop complete conviction and faith, it is very difficult for them to continue in Kṛṣṇa consciousness. We have practical experience in discharging our missionary activity that some people come and apply themselves to Kṛṣṇa consciousness with some hidden motive, and as soon as they are economically a little well situated, they give up this process and take to their old ways again. It is only by faith that one can advance in Kṛṣṇa consciousness.

As far as the development of faith is concerned, one who is well versed in the literatures of devotional service and has attained the stage of firm faith is called a first-class person in Kṛṣṇa consciousness. And in the second class are those who are not very advanced in understanding the devotional scriptures but who automatically have firm faith that *kṛṣṇa-bhakti*, or service to Kṛṣṇa, is the best course and so in good faith have taken it up. Thus they are superior to the third class, who have neither perfect knowledge of the scriptures nor good faith but by association and simplicity are trying to follow. The third-class person in Kṛṣṇa consciousness may fall down, but when one is in the second-class or first-class position, he does not fall down. The first-class devotee will surely make progress and achieve the result at the end. As far as the third-class person in Kṛṣṇa consciousness is concerned, although he has the conviction that devotional service to Kṛṣṇa is very good, he has no knowledge of Kṛṣṇa from scriptures like *Śrīmad-Bhāgavatam* and the *Bhagavad-gītā*. Sometimes these third-class persons in Kṛṣṇa consciousness have some tendency toward *karma-yoga* and *jñāna-yoga*, and sometimes they are disturbed, but as soon as the infection of *karma-yoga* or *jñāna-yoga* is vanquished, they become second-class or first-class persons in Kṛṣṇa consciousness. Faith in Kṛṣṇa is also divided into three stages and described in *Śrīmad-Bhāgavatam.* First-class attachment, second-class attachment, and third-class attachment are also explained in *Śrīmad-Bhāgavatam,* in the Eleventh Canto.

However one is situated, one should have the determination to go out and preach Kṛṣṇa consciousness. That endeavor should at least be there, and one who attempts to preach renders the best service to the Lord. Despite opposition, one should attempt to elevate people to the highest standard of self-realization. One who has actually seen the truth, who is in the trance of self-realization, cannot just sit idly. He must go out. Rāmānujācārya, for instance, publicly declared the *mantra* his spiritual master had given him. He did not distribute it secretly for some fee. Recently, an Indian *yogī* came to America to give some "private *mantra.*" But if a *mantra* has any power, why should it be private? If a *mantra* is powerful, why should it not be publicly declared so that everyone can take advantage of it? We are saying that this Hare Kṛṣṇa *mahā-mantra* can save everyone, and we are therefore distributing it publicly, free of charge. But in this age, people are so foolish that they are not prepared to accept it. Rather, they hanker after some secret *mantra* and therefore pay some "*yogī*" thirty-five dollars or whatever for some "private *mantra.*" This is because people want to be cheated. But the devotees are preaching without charge, declaring in the streets, parks, and everywhere, "Here! Here is the Hare Kṛṣṇa *mahā-mantra.* Come on, take it!" But under the spell of *māyā,* illusion, people are thinking, "Oh, this is not good." But if you charge something and bluff and cheat people, they will follow you.

In this regard, there is a Hindi verse stating that Kali-yuga is such an abominable age that if one speaks the truth people will come and beat him, but if one cheats, bluffs, and lies people will be bewildered, will like it, and will accept it. If I say, "I am God," people will say, "Oh, here is Swāmījī. Here is God." In this age, people don't have sufficient brain power to inquire, "How have you become God? What are the symptoms of God?

Do you have all these symptoms?" Because people do not make such inquiries, they are cheated. Therefore it is necessary to be fixed in consciousness of the Self. Unless one knows and understands the real self and the Superself, one will be cheated. Real *yoga* means understanding this process of self-realization.

> *yato yato niścalati manaś cañcalam asthiram*
> *tatas tato niyamyaitad ātmany eva vaśaṁ nayet*

"From whatever and wherever the mind wanders due to its flickering and unsteady nature, one must certainly withdraw it and bring it back under the control of the Self." (Bg. 6.26) This is the real yogic process. If you are trying to concentrate your mind on Kṛṣṇa and the mind is diverted—wandering to some cinema or wherever—you should withdraw the mind, thinking, "Not there, please. Here." This is *yoga:* not allowing the mind to wander from Kṛṣṇa.

Very intense training is required to keep the mind fixed on Kṛṣṇa while sitting in one place. That is very hard work indeed. If one is not so practiced and tries to imitate this process, he will surely be confused. Instead, we always have to engage ourselves in Kṛṣṇa consciousness, dovetailing everything we do to Kṛṣṇa. Our usual activities should be so molded that they are rendered for Kṛṣṇa's sake. In this way the mind will remain fixed on Kṛṣṇa. As stated before, we should not try to sit down and stare at the tip of our nose. At the present moment, attempts to engage in that type of *yoga* are artificial. Rather, the recommended method is chanting the Hare Kṛṣṇa *mantra* loudly and hearing it. Then, even if the mind is diverted, it will be forced to concentrate on the sound vibration "Hare Kṛṣṇa." It isn't necessary to withdraw the mind from everything; it will automatically be withdrawn, because it will be concentrated on the sound vibration. If we hear an automobile pass, our attention is automatically diverted. Similarly, if we constantly chant Hare Kṛṣṇa, our mind will automatically be fixed on Kṛṣṇa, although we are accustomed to thinking of so many other things.

The nature of the mind is flickering and unsteady. But a self-realized *yogī* has to control the mind; the mind should not control him. At the present moment, the mind is controlling us (*go-*

dāsa). The mind is telling us, "Please, why not look at that beautiful girl?" and so we look. It says, "Why not drink that nice liquor?" and we say, "Yes." It says, "Why not smoke this cigarette?" "Yes," we say. "Why not go to this restaurant for such palatable food? Why not do this? Why not do that?" In this way the mind is dictating and we are following. Material life means being controlled by the senses, or by the mind, which is the center of all the senses. Being controlled by the mind means being controlled by the senses, because the senses are the mind's assistants. The master mind dictates, "Go see that," and the eyes, following the directions of the mind, look at the sense object. The mind tells us to go to a certain place, and the legs, under the mind's directions, carry us there. Thus, being under the direction of the mind means coming under the control of the senses. If we can control the mind, we will not be under the control of the senses. One who is under the control of the senses is known as *go-dāsa.* The word *go* means "senses," and *dāsa* means "servant." One who is the master of his senses is called a *gosvāmī,* because *svāmī* means "master." Therefore, one who has the title *gosvāmī* is one who has mastered his senses. As long as one is the servant of his senses, he cannot be called a *gosvāmī* or *svāmī.* Unless one masters his senses, his acceptance of the title *svāmī* or *gosvāmī* is just a form of cheating. It was Rūpa Gosvāmī who thus defined the meaning of the word *gosvāmī.* Originally, Sanātana Gosvāmī and Rūpa Gosvāmī were not *gosvāmīs* but were government ministers. It was only when they became disciples of Lord Caitanya Mahāprabhu that they became *gosvāmīs.* So *gosvāmī* is not a hereditary title but a qualification. One becomes so qualified under the directions of a bona fide spiritual master. Only when one has attained perfection in sense control can he be called a *gosvāmī* and become a spiritual master in his turn. Unless one can master the senses, he will simply be a bogus spiritual master.

Rūpa Gosvāmī explains this in his *Upadeśāmṛta* (1):

vāco vegaṁ manasaḥ krodha-vegaṁ
jihvā-vegam udaropastha-vegam
etān vegān yo viṣaheta dhīraḥ
sarvām apīmāṁ pṛthivīṁ sa śiṣyāt

"A sober person who can tolerate the urge to speak, the mind's demands, the actions of anger, and the urges of the tongue, belly, and genitals is qualified to make disciples all over the world." In this verse Rūpa Gosvāmī mentions six "pushings" (*vegas*). A pushing is a kind of impetus. For instance, when nature calls, we have to go to the toilet, and we cannot check this urge. So this urge is called a *vega,* a kind of pushing. According to Rūpa Gosvāmī, there are six *vegas. Vāco vega* is the urge to talk unnecessarily. That is a kind of pushing of the tongue. Then there is *krodha-vega,* the urge to become angry. When we are pushed to anger, we cannot check ourselves, and sometimes men become so angry that they commit murder. Similarly, the mind is pushing, dictating, "You must go there at once," and we immediately go where we are told. The word *jihvā-vega* refers to the tongue's being urged to taste palatable foods. *Udara-vega* refers to the urges of the belly. Although the belly is full, it still wants more food, and that is a kind of pushing of the belly. And when we yield to the pushings of the tongue and the belly, the urges of the genitals become very strong, and sex is required. If one does not control his mind or his tongue, how can he control his genitals? In this way, there are so many pushings, so much so that the body is a kind of pushing machine. Rūpa Gosvāmī therefore tells us that one can become a spiritual master only when he can control all these urges.

Etān vegān yo viṣaheta dhīraḥ sarvām apīmāṁ pṛthivīṁ sa śiṣyāt: "One who can control the pushings and remain steady can make disciples all over the world." The word *dhīra* means "steady, sober." Only one who is *dhīra* is qualified to make disciples. This all depends on one's training. Indeed, *yoga* means training the mind and the senses to be fixed on the Self. This is not possible by meditating only fifteen minutes a day and then going out and doing whatever the senses dictate. How can the problems of life be solved so cheaply? If we want something precious, we have to pay for it. By the grace of Lord Caitanya, this payment has been made very easy—just chant Hare Kṛṣṇa. By our chanting, this system of control, this *yoga* system, becomes perfected. *Ihā haite sarva siddhi haibe tomāra.* Thus Lord Caitanya has blessed us. Simply by chanting Hare Kṛṣṇa, we will achieve the perfection of self-realization. In this Age of Kali, when people are so fallen, other processes will not be successful. This is the only process, and it is easy, sublime, effective, and practical. By it, one can realize oneself.

According to Kṛṣṇa in the Ninth Chapter of the *Bhagavad-gītā* (9.2), this process is the most sublime.

rāja-vidyā rāja-guhyaṁ pavitram idam uttamam
pratyakṣāvagamaṁ dharmyaṁ su-sukhaṁ kartum avyayam

"This knowledge is the king of education, the most secret of all secrets. It is the purest knowledge, and because it gives direct perception of the self by realization, it is the perfection of religion. It is everlasting, and it is joyfully performed."

After eating, a man can understand that his hunger has been satisfied; similarly, by following the principles of Kṛṣṇa consciousness, one can understand that he is advancing in self-realization.

6
Perception of the Supersoul

praśānta-manasaṁ hy enaṁ yoginaṁ sukham uttamam
upaiti śānta-rajasaṁ brahma-bhūtam akalmaṣam

"The *yogī* whose mind is fixed on Me verily attains the highest perfection of transcendental happiness. He is beyond the mode of passion, he realizes his qualitative identity with the Supreme, and thus he is freed from all reactions to past deeds." (Bg. 6.27)

yuñjann evaṁ sadātmānaṁ yogī vigata-kalmaṣaḥ
sukhena brahma-saṁsparśam atyantaṁ sukham aśnute

"Thus the self-controlled *yogī*, constantly engaged in *yoga* practice, becomes free from all material contamination and achieves the highest stage of perfect happiness in transcendental loving service to the Lord." (Bg. 6.28)

So here is the perfection: "The *yogī* whose mind is fixed on Me . . ." Since Kṛṣṇa is speaking, "Me" means Kṛṣṇa. If I say, "Give me a glass of water," I do not intend that the water should be supplied to someone else. We must therefore clearly understand that, since the *Bhagavad-gītā* is being spoken by Śrī Kṛṣṇa, when He says "unto Me," He means unto Kṛṣṇa. Unfortunately, there are many commentators who deviate from these clear instructions. I do not know why; their motives are no doubt nefarious.

sarva-bhūta-stham ātmānaṁ sarva-bhūtāni cātmani
īkṣate yoga-yuktātmā sarvatra sama-darśanaḥ

"A true *yogī* observes Me in all beings and also sees every being in Me. Indeed, the self-realized person sees Me, the same Supreme Lord, everywhere." (Bg. 6.29) *Sarva-bhūta-stham ātmānam:* "A true *yogī* observes Me in all beings." How is this possible? Some people say that all beings are Kṛṣṇa and that therefore there is no point in worshiping Kṛṣṇa separately. Consequently, such people take to humanitarian activities, claiming that such work is better. They say, "Why should Kṛṣṇa be worshiped? Kṛṣṇa says that one should see Kṛṣṇa in every being. Therefore let us serve *daridra-nārāyaṇa*, the man in the street." Such misinterpreters do not know the proper techniques of serving Kṛṣṇa in all beings, which have to be learned under a bona fide spiritual master.

A true *yogī*, as explained before, is the devotee of Kṛṣṇa, and the most advanced devotee goes forth to preach Kṛṣṇa consciousness. Why? Because he sees Kṛṣṇa in all beings. How is this? Because he sees that all beings are part and parcel of Kṛṣṇa. He also understands that since these beings have forgotten Kṛṣṇa it is his duty to awaken them to Kṛṣṇa consciousness. Sometimes missionaries go forth to educate primitive, uneducated people just because they see that they are human beings and so deserve to be educated in order to understand the value of life. This is due to the missionary's sympathy. The devotee is similarly motivated. He understands that everyone should know himself to be part and parcel of Kṛṣṇa. The devotee understands that people are suffering due to their forgetfulness of Kṛṣṇa.

Thus the devotee sees Kṛṣṇa in everything. He is not under the illusion that everything has become Kṛṣṇa. Rather, he sees every living being as the son of God. If I say that this boy is the son of Mr. Johnson, do I mean that this boy is Mr. Johnson himself? I may see Mr. Johnson in this boy because this boy is his son, but the distinction remains. If I see every living being as the son of Kṛṣṇa, I see Kṛṣṇa in every being. This should not be difficult to understand. It is neither an association nor a vision but a fact.

When a devotee sees a cat or a dog, he sees Kṛṣṇa in him. He knows that a cat, for instance, is a living being and that due to his past deeds he has received the body of a cat. This is due to his forgetfulness. The devotee helps the cat by giving it some *kṛṣṇa-prasādam* so that someday the cat will come to Kṛṣṇa consciousness. This is seeing Kṛṣṇa in the cat. The devotee does not think, "Oh, here is Kṛṣṇa. Let me embrace this cat and serve this cat as God." Such thinking is nonsensical. If one sees a tiger, he does not say, "Oh, here is Kṛṣṇa. Come on, please eat me." The devotee does not embrace all beings as Kṛṣṇa but rather sympathizes with every living being because he sees all beings as part and parcel of Kṛṣṇa. In this way, "the true *yogī* observes Me in all beings." This is real vision.

Whatever is done in Kṛṣṇa consciousness, knowingly or unknowingly, will have its effect. Children who bow down or try to vibrate Kṛṣṇa's names or clap during *kīrtana* are actually accumulating so much in their bank account of Kṛṣṇa consciousness. Fire will act, whether one is a child or an adult. If a child touches fire, the fire will burn. The fire does not say, "Oh, I will not burn him. He is a child and does not know." No, the fire will always act as fire. Similarly, Kṛṣṇa is the supreme spirit, and if a child partakes in Kṛṣṇa consciousness, he will be affected. Kṛṣṇa will act, whether the child knows or does not know. Every living being should be given a chance to partake in Kṛṣṇa consciousness because Kṛṣṇa is there and will act. Therefore everyone is being invited to come and take *prasādam*, because this *prasādam* will someday take effect.

We should be careful not to make the mistake of thinking that everyone is Kṛṣṇa; rather, we should see Kṛṣṇa in everyone. Kṛṣṇa is all-pervading. Why is He to be seen only in human beings? As stated in the *Brahma-saṁhitā*, He is also present within the atom: *aṇḍāntara-stha-paramāṇu-cayāntara-stham.* The word *paramāṇu* means "atom," and we should understand that Kṛṣṇa is present within every atom. "A true *yogī* observes Me in all beings and also sees every being in Me." How does the *yogī* see every being "in Me"? This is possible because the true *yogī* knows that everything that we see is Kṛṣṇa. We may sit on a floor or on a carpet, but in actuality we are sitting on Kṛṣṇa. We should know this to be a fact. How is a carpet Kṛṣṇa? It is Kṛṣṇa because it is made of Kṛṣṇa's energy. The Supreme Lord has various energies, of which there are three primary divisions—the material energy, the spiritual energy, and the marginal energy. *Parāsya śaktir vividhaiva śrūyate.* We living entities are the marginal energy, the material world is the material energy, and the spiritual world is the spiritual energy. We are marginal in the sense that we can be either spiritually or materially situated. There is no third alternative: either we become materialistic or spiritualistic.

As long as we are in the material world, we are seated on the material energy, and therefore we are situated in Kṛṣṇa, because Kṛṣṇa's energy is not separate from Kṛṣṇa. A flame contains both heat and illumination, two energies. Neither the heat nor the illumination is separate from the flame; therefore in one sense heat is fire, and illumination is fire, but they can be distinguished. Similarly, the material energy is also Kṛṣṇa, and although we may think we are sitting on a floor, we are actually sitting on Kṛṣṇa. Therefore it is stated, "The self-realized man sees Me everywhere." Seeing Kṛṣṇa everywhere means seeing every living being as well as everything else in relationship to Kṛṣṇa. In the Seventh Chapter of the *Bhagavad-gītā* (7.8), Lord Kṛṣṇa tells Arjuna how He can be seen in various manifestations.

raso 'ham apsu kaunteya prabhāsmi śaśi-sūryayoḥ
praṇavaḥ sarva-vedeṣu śabdaḥ khe pauruṣaṁ nṛṣu

"O son of Kuntī, I am the taste of water, the light of the sun and the moon, the syllable *oṁ* in the Vedic *mantras;* I am the sound in ether and ability in man."

Water is drunk by all living entities; it is needed by birds, beasts, and man. It is used not only for drinking but for washing and for cultivating plants as well. A soldier on the battlefield can understand how important water is. When fighting, soldiers become thirsty, and if they have no water, they die. Once a person has learned the philosophy of the *Bhagavad-gītā*, whenever he drinks water he sees Kṛṣṇa. And when does a day pass when we do not drink water? This is the way of Kṛṣṇa consciousness. "I am the light of the sun and the moon." So whether in the day or the night, we see either sunshine or moonshine. How, then, can we forget Kṛṣṇa? This, then, is the way of perfect *yoga.* We have to see Kṛṣṇa everywhere and at all times.

yo māṁ paśyati sarvatra sarvaṁ ca mayi paśyati
tasyāhaṁ na praṇaśyāmi sa ca me na praṇaśyati

"For one who sees Me everywhere and sees everything in Me, I am never lost, nor is he ever lost to Me." (Bg. 6.30) This is *sadā tad-bhāva-bhāvitaḥ:* always remembering Kṛṣṇa. If we practice living in this way, we never lose Kṛṣṇa and are never lost to Kṛṣṇa, and at the time of death we are therefore sure to go to Kṛṣṇa. If we are not lost to Kṛṣṇa, where can we go but to Kṛṣṇa? In the Ninth Chapter Kṛṣṇa tells Arjuna, *kaunteya pratijānīhi na me bhaktaḥ praṇaśyati* (Bg. 9.31): "O son of Kuntī, declare it boldly that My devotee never perishes."

Simply don't lose sight of Kṛṣṇa. That is the perfection of life. We can forget everything else, but we should never forget Kṛṣṇa. If we can remember Kṛṣṇa we are the richest of men, even though people may see us as very poor. Although Rūpa Gosvāmī and Sanātana Gosvāmī had been learned scholars and very opulent ministers, they adopted the poor life of mendicants. In his *Śrī Ṣaḍ-gosvāmy-aṣṭaka* (verse 4), Śrīnivāsa Ācārya thus describes the six Gosvāmīs:

tyaktvā tūrṇam aśeṣa-maṇḍala-pati-śreṇīṁ sadā tuccha-vat
bhūtvā dīna-gaṇeśakau karuṇayā kaupīna-kanthāśritau
gopī-bhāva-rasāmṛtābdhi-laharī-kallola-magnau muhur
vande rūpa-sanātanau raghu-yugau śrī-jīva-gopālakau

"I offer my respectful obeisances unto the six Gosvāmīs—Śrī Rūpa Gosvāmī, Śrī Sanātana Gosvāmī, Śrī Raghunātha Bhaṭṭa Gosvāmī, Śrī Raghunātha dāsa Gosvāmī, Śrī Jīva Gosvāmī, and Śrī Gopāla Bhaṭṭa Gosvāmī—who cast off all aristocratic association as insignificant. To deliver the poor, conditioned souls, they accepted loincloths and became mendicants, but they were always merged in the ecstatic ocean of the *gopīs'* love for Kṛṣṇa, and they were always bathing repeatedly in the waves of that ocean."

The words *kaupīna-kanthāśritau* indicate that the Gosvāmīs were simply wearing underwear and a loincloth and nothing else. In other words, they accepted the poorest way of life as mendicants. Generally, one who is habituated to living according to a high standard cannot immediately lower his standard. In other words, a rich man who is forced to accept a poor condition generally cannot live. But the Gosvāmīs lived very happily. How was this possible? *Gopī-bhāva-rasāmṛtābdhi-laharī-kallola-magnau muhur.* They were actually rich because they were constantly dipping themselves in the ocean of the loving affairs of the *gopīs.* If one simply thinks of Kṛṣṇa's loving exchanges with the *gopīs,* one is not lost. There are many ways not to lose sight of Kṛṣṇa. If we do not lose sight of Kṛṣṇa, then we will not be lost.

A person in Kṛṣṇa consciousness certainly sees Lord Kṛṣṇa everywhere, and he sees everything in Kṛṣṇa. Such a person may appear to see all separate manifestations of the material nature, but in each and every instance he is conscious of Kṛṣṇa, knowing that everything is the manifestation of Kṛṣṇa's energy. Nothing can exist without Kṛṣṇa, and Kṛṣṇa is the Lord of everything—this is the basic principle of Kṛṣṇa consciousness. How does the devotee know that everything is the manifestation of Kṛṣṇa's energy? First of all, a Kṛṣṇa conscious person is a philosopher. If he sees a tree, he thinks, "What is this tree?" He then sees that the tree has a material body—just as he has a material body—and that the tree is also a living entity. He also sees that due to the living entity's past misdeeds he has obtained such an abominable body that he cannot even move. The tree's body is material, material energy, and the devotee automatically questions, "Whose energy? Kṛṣṇa's energy. Therefore the tree is connected to Kṛṣṇa. Being a living entity, the tree is part and parcel of Kṛṣṇa." In this way the Kṛṣṇa conscious person does not see the tree but sees Kṛṣṇa present. That is Kṛṣṇa consciousness: you don't see the tree, you see Kṛṣṇa. That is the perfection of *yoga*, and that is also *samādhi.*

Kṛṣṇa consciousness is the development of love of Kṛṣṇa—a position transcendental even to material liberation. Why does the Kṛṣṇa conscious person take such an account of a tree? Because he has love for Kṛṣṇa. If you love your child and your child is away, you think of him when you see his shoe. You think, "Oh, this is my dear child's shoe." It is not that you love the shoe; you love the child. The shoe, however, evokes that love. Similarly, as soon as we see Kṛṣṇa's energy manifested in a living entity, we love that entity because we love Kṛṣṇa. Therefore, if we love Kṛṣṇa, universal love is accounted for. Otherwise "universal love" is nonsensical, because it is not possible to love everybody without loving Kṛṣṇa. If we love Kṛṣṇa, universal love is automatically there. Without being Kṛṣṇa conscious, a person may say, "Here is my American brother, and here is my Indian brother. Now let us eat this cow." Such a person may look on other humans as brothers, but he looks on the cow as food. Is this universal love? A Kṛṣṇa conscious person, however, thinks, "Oh, here is a cow. Here is a dog. They are part and parcel of Kṛṣṇa, but somehow or other they have acquired different bodies. This does not mean that they are not my brothers. How can I kill and eat my brothers?" That is true universal love—rooted in love for Kṛṣṇa. Without such Kṛṣṇa consciousness, there is no question of love at all.

Kṛṣṇa consciousness is the stage beyond self-realization in which the devotee becomes one with Kṛṣṇa in the sense that Kṛṣṇa becomes everything for the devotee and the devotee becomes full in loving Kṛṣṇa. An intimate relationship between the Lord and the devotee then exists. In that stage, the living entity attains his immortality. Nor is the Personality of Godhead ever out of sight of the devotee. To merge in Kṛṣṇa is spiritual annihilation. A devotee takes no such risk. It is stated in the *Brahma-saṁhitā* (5.38),

premāñjana-cchurita-bhakti-vilocanena
santaḥ sadaiva hṛdayeṣu vilokayanti
yaṁ śyāmasundaram acintya-guṇa-svarūpaṁ
govindam ādi-puruṣaṁ tam ahaṁ bhajāmi

"I worship Govinda, the primeval Lord, who is Śyāmasundara, Kṛṣṇa Himself with inconceivable innumerable attributes, whom the pure devotees see in their heart of hearts with the eye of devotion tinged with the salve of love." One who has developed such a love for Kṛṣṇa sees Śyāmasundara, Kartāmeśāna, always within his heart. At this stage Lord Kṛṣṇa never disappears from the sight of the devotee, nor does the devotee ever lose sight of the Lord. In the case of a *yogī* who sees the Lord as the Paramātmā within the heart, the same applies. Such a *yogī* turns into a pure devotee and cannot bear to live for a moment without seeing the Lord within himself.

This is the real process by which we can see God. God is not our order-supplier. We cannot demand, "Come and show Yourself." No, we first have to qualify ourselves. Then we can see God at every moment and everywhere.

sarva-bhūta-sthitaṁ yo māṁ bhajaty ekatvam āsthitaḥ
sarvathā vartamāno 'pi sa yogī mayi vartate

"Such a *yogī*, who engages in the worshipful service of the Supersoul, knowing that I and the Supersoul are one, remains always in Me in all circumstances." (Bg. 6.31)

A *yogī* who is practicing meditation on the Supersoul sees within himself the plenary portion of Kṛṣṇa as Viṣṇu—with four hands, holding conchshell, wheel, club, and lotus flower. This manifestation of Viṣṇu, which is the *yogī's* object of concentration, is Kṛṣṇa's plenary portion. As stated in *Brahma-saṁhitā* (5.48),

yasyaika-niśvasita-kālam athāvalambya
jīvanti loma-vilajā jagad-aṇḍa-nāthāḥ
viṣṇur mahān sa iha yasya kalā-viśeṣo
govindam ādi-puruṣaṁ tam ahaṁ bhajāmi

"The Brahmās and other lords of the mundane worlds appear from the pores of Mahā-Viṣṇu and remain alive for the duration of His one exhalation. I adore the primeval Lord, Govinda, of whom Mahā-Viṣṇu is a portion of a plenary portion." The words *govindam ādi-puruṣaṁ tam ahaṁ bhajāmi* ("I worship Govinda, the primeval Lord") are most important. The word *ādi* means "original," and *puruṣam* means "the Lord as the original male, the original enjoyer." And who is this Govinda whose plenary portion is Mahā-Viṣṇu? And what is the function of Mahā-Viṣṇu?

In every universe there is a primary, original living entity known as Brahmā. The life of Brahmā is the life of the universe, and this life exists during only one breathing period (exhalation and inhalation) of Mahā-Viṣṇu. Mahā-Viṣṇu lies on the Causal Ocean, and when He exhales, millions of universes issue from His body as bubbles and then develop. When Mahā-Viṣṇu inhales, these millions of universes return within Him, and this is called the process of annihilation. That, in essence, is the position of these material universes: they come out from the body of Mahā-Viṣṇu and then again return. In the Ninth Chapter of the *Bhagavad-gītā* (9.7) it is confirmed that the material universes are manifested at a certain period and are then annihilated.

sarva-bhūtāni kaunteya prakṛtiṁ yānti māmikām
kalpa-kṣaye punas tāni kalpādau visṛjāmy aham

"O son of Kuntī, at the end of the millennium all material manifestations enter into My nature, and at the beginning of another millennium, by My potency, I create them again." The creation, maintenance, and annihilation of the material cosmic manifestation are completely dependent on the supreme will of the Personality of Godhead. "At the end of the millennium" means at the death of Brahmā. Brahmā lives for one hundred years, and his one day is calculated at 4,320,000,000 of our earthly years. His night is of the same duration. His month consists of thirty such days and nights, and his year of twelve months. After one hundred such years, when Brahmā dies, the devastation or annihilation takes place; this means that the energy manifested by the Supreme Lord is again wound up in Himself. That is, Mahā-Viṣṇu inhales. Then again, when there is a need to manifest the cosmic world, it is done by His will: "Although I am one, I shall become many." This is the Vedic aphorism. He expands Himself in this material energy, and the whole cosmic manifestation again takes place.

Since the entire creation and annihilation of the material universes depend on the exhaling and inhaling of Mahā-Viṣṇu, we can hardly imagine the magnitude of Mahā-Viṣṇu. And yet it is said here that Mahā-Viṣṇu is but a plenary portion of the plenary portion of Kṛṣṇa, who is the original Govinda. Mahā-Viṣṇu enters into each universe as Garbhodakaśāyī Viṣṇu, and Garbhodakaśāyī Viṣṇu further expands as Kṣīrodakaśāyī Viṣṇu, and it is this Viṣṇu form that enters into the heart of every living entity. In this way, Viṣṇu is manifested throughout the creation. Thus the *yogīs* concentrate their minds on the Kṣīrodakaśāyī Viṣṇu form within the heart. As stated in the last chapter of the *Bhagavad-gītā* (18.61),

īśvaraḥ sarva-bhūtānāṁ hṛd-deśe 'rjuna tiṣṭhati
bhrāmayan sarva-bhūtāni yantrārūḍhāni māyayā

"The Supreme Lord is situated in everyone's heart, O Arjuna, and is directing the wanderings of all living entities, who are seated as on a machine made of the material energy."

Thus, according to the yogic process, the *yogī* finds out where Kṣīrodakaśāyī Viṣṇu is seated within his heart, and when he finds this form there, he concentrates on Him. The *yogī* should know that this Viṣṇu is not different from Kṛṣṇa. Kṛṣṇa in this form of Supersoul is situated in everyone's heart. Furthermore, there is no difference between the innumerable Supersouls present in the innumerable hearts of the living entities. For example, there is only one sun in the sky, but this sun may be reflected in millions of buckets of water. Or, one may ask millions of people, "Where is the sun?" and each person will say, "Over my head." The sun is one, but it is reflected countless times. According to the *Vedas*, the living entities are innumerable; there is no possibility of counting them. Just as the sun can be reflected in countless buckets of water, Viṣṇu, the Supreme Personality of Godhead, can live in everyone's heart. It is this form that is Kṛṣṇa's plenary portion, and it is this form on which the *yogī* concentrates.

One who is engaged in Kṛṣṇa consciousness is already a perfect *yogī*. In fact, there is no difference between a Kṛṣṇa conscious devotee always engaged in the transcendental loving service of Kṛṣṇa and a perfect *yogī* engaged in meditation on the Supersoul. There is no difference between a *yogī* in *samādhi* (in a trance meditating on the Viṣṇu form) and a Kṛṣṇa conscious person engaged in different activities. The devotee—even though engaged in various activities while in material existence—remains always situated in Kṛṣṇa. This is confirmed in the *Bhakti-rasāmṛta-sindhu* of Śrīla Rūpa Gosvāmī: *nikhilāsv apy avasthāsu jīvan-muktaḥ sa ucyate*. A devotee of the Lord, always acting in Kṛṣṇa consciousness, is automatically liberated. This is also confirmed in the Fourteenth Chapter of the *Bhagavad-gītā* (14.26):

māṁ ca yo 'vyabhicāreṇa bhakti-yogena sevate
sa guṇān samatītyaitān brahma-bhūyāya kalpate

"One who engages in full devotional service, unfailing in all circumstances, at once transcends the modes of material nature and thus comes to the level of Brahman."

Thus the devotee engaged in unalloyed devotional service has already transcended the material modes of nature. Being situated on the Brahman platform means being liberated. There are three platforms: the bodily, or sensual; the mental; and the spiritual. The spiritual platform is called the Brahman platform, and liberation means being situated on that platform. Being conditioned souls, we are presently situated on the bodily, or sensual, platform. Those who are a little advanced—speculators, philosophers—are situated on the mental platform. Above this is the platform of liberation, of Brahman realization.

That the devotee who always acts in Kṛṣṇa consciousness is automatically situated on the liberated platform of Brahman is confirmed in the *Nārada-pañcarātra:*

dik-kālādy-anavacchinne kṛṣṇe ceto vidhāya ca
tan-mayo bhavati kṣipraṁ jīvo brahmaṇi yojayet

"By concentrating one's attention on the transcendental form of Kṛṣṇa, who is all-pervading and beyond time and space, one becomes absorbed in thinking of Kṛṣṇa and then attains the happy state of transcendental association with Him."

Kṛṣṇa consciousness is the highest stage of trance in *yoga* practice. This very understanding that Kṛṣṇa is present as the Paramātmā in everyone's heart makes the *yogī* faultless. The *Vedas* confirm this inconceivable potency of the Lord as follows:

eka eva paro viṣṇuḥ sarva-vyāpī na saṁśayaḥ
aiśvaryād rūpam ekaṁ ca sūrya-vat bahudheyate

"Viṣṇu is one, and yet He is certainly all-pervading. By His inconceivable potency, in spite of His one form, He is present everywhere, as the sun appears in many places at once."

ātmaupamyena sarvatra samaṁ paśyati yo 'rjuna
sukhaṁ vā yadi vā duḥkhaṁ sa yogī paramo mataḥ

"He is a perfect *yogī* who, by comparison with his own self, sees the true equality of all beings, both in their happiness and distress, O Arjuna!" (Bg. 6.32) This is true universal vision. It is not that God is sitting in my heart and not in the heart of a dog, cat, or cow. *Sarva-bhūtānām* means that He is sitting in the hearts of all living entities, in the human heart and in the ant's heart. The only difference is that cats and dogs cannot realize this. A human being, if he tries to follow the *sāṅkhya-yoga* or *bhakti-yoga* system, is able to understand, and this is the prerogative of human life. We have undergone the evolutionary process and have passed through more than eight million species of life in order to get this human form, and therefore if we miss this opportunity we suffer a great loss. We should be conscious of this and careful not to miss this opportunity. We have a good body, the human form, and intelligence and civilization. We should not live like animals and struggle hard for existence but should utilize our time thinking peacefully and understanding our relationship with the Supreme Lord. This is the instruction of the *Bhagavad-gītā:* Don't lose this opportunity; utilize it properly.

7
Yoga for the Modern Age

arjuna uvāca
yo 'yaṁ yogas tvayā proktaḥ sāmyena madhusūdana
etasyāhaṁ na paśyāmi cañcalatvāt sthitiṁ sthirām

"Arjuna said, 'O Madhusūdana, the system of *yoga* You have summarized appears impractical and unendurable to me, for the mind is restless and unsteady.'" (Bg. 6.33)

This is the crucial test of the eightfold *aṣṭāṅga-yoga* system expounded herein by Lord Śrī Kṛṣṇa. It has already been explained that one must sit in a certain way and concentrate the mind on the form of Viṣṇu seated within the heart. According to the *aṣṭāṅga-yoga* system, first of all one has to control the senses, follow all the rules and regulations, practice the sitting posture and the breathing process, concentrate the mind on the form of Viṣṇu within the heart, and then become absorbed in that form. There are eight processes in this *aṣṭāṅga-yoga* system, but herein Arjuna says quite frankly that this *aṣṭāṅga-yoga* system is very difficult. Indeed, he says that it "appears impractical and unendurable to me."

Actually, the *aṣṭāṅga-yoga* system is not impractical, for were it impractical Lord Kṛṣṇa would not have taken so much trouble to describe it. It is not impractical, but it *appears* impractical. What may be impractical for one man may be practical for another. Arjuna is a representative of the common man in the sense that he is not a mendicant or a *sannyāsī* or a scholar. He is on the battlefield fighting for his kingdom, and in this sense he is an ordinary man engaged in a worldly activity. He is concerned with earning a livelihood, supporting his family, and so on. Arjuna has many problems, just as the common man, and generally this system of *aṣṭāṅga-yoga* is impractical for the ordinary common man. That is the point being made. It is practical for one who has already completely renounced everything and can sit in a secluded, sacred place in a forest or cave. But who can do this in this age? Although Arjuna was a great warrior, a member of the royal family, and a very advanced person, he proclaims this *yoga* system impractical. And what are we in comparison to Arjuna? If we attempt this system, failure is certain.

Therefore the system of mysticism described by Lord Kṛṣṇa to Arjuna in the Sixth Chapter of the *Bhagavad-gītā*—beginning with the words *śucau deśe* and ending with *yogī paramaḥ*—is here rejected by Arjuna out of a feeling of inability. As stated before, it is not possible for an ordinary man to leave home and go to a secluded place in the mountains or jungles to practice *yoga* in this Age of Kali. The present age is characterized by a bitter struggle for a life of short duration. As Kali-yuga progresses, our life span gets shorter and shorter. Our forefathers lived for a hundred years or more, but now people are dying at the age of sixty or seventy. Gradually the life span will decrease even further. Memory, mercy, and other good qualities will also decrease in this age.

In Kali-yuga, people are not serious about self-realization even by simple, practical means, and what to speak of this difficult *yoga* system, which regulates the mode of living, the manner of sitting, selection of place, and detachment of the mind from material engagements. As a practical man, Arjuna thought it was impossible to follow this system of *yoga*, even though he was favorably endowed in many ways. He was not prepared to become a pseudo *yogī* and practice some gymnastic feats. He was not a pretender but a soldier and a family man. Therefore he frankly admitted that for him this system of *yoga* would be a waste of time. Arjuna belonged to the royal family and was highly elevated in terms of numerous qualities; he was a great warrior, he had great longevity, and, above all, he was the most intimate friend of Lord Kṛṣṇa, the Supreme Personality of Godhead. Five thousand years ago, when Arjuna was living, the life span was very long. At that time people used to live up to one thousand years. In the present age, Kali-yuga, the life span is limited to a hundred years, in Dvāpara-yuga the life span was a thousand years, in Tretā-yuga the life span was ten thousand years, and in Satya-yuga the life span was one hundred thousand years. Thus as the *yugas* degenerate, the life span decreases. Even though Arjuna was living at a time when one could live and practice meditation for a thousand years, he still considered this system impossible.

Five thousand years ago, Arjuna had much better facilities than we do now, yet he refused to accept this system of *yoga*. In fact, we do not find any record in history of his practicing it at any time. Therefore, this system must be considered generally impossible in this Age of Kali. Of course, it may be possible for some very few, rare men, but for the people in general it is an impossible proposal. If this were so five thousand years ago, what of the present day? Those who are imitating this *yoga* system in different so-called schools and societies, although complacent, are certainly wasting their time. They are completely ignorant of the desired goal.

Since the *aṣṭāṅga-yoga* system is considered impossible, the *bhakti-yoga* system is recommended for everyone. Without training or education, one can automatically participate in *bhakti-yoga*. Even a small child can clap at *kīrtana*. Therefore Lord Caitanya Mahāprabhu has proclaimed *bhakti-yoga* the only system practical for this age.

harer nāma harer nāma harer nāmaiva kevalam
kalau nāsty eva nāsty eva nāsty eva gatir anyathā

"In this age of quarrel and hypocrisy, the only means of deliverance is chanting the holy name of the Lord. There is no other way. There is no other way. There is no other way." Chanting is very simple, and one will feel the results immediately. *Pratyakṣāvagamaṁ dharmyam.* If we attempt to practice other *yoga* systems, we will remain in darkness; we will not know whether or not we are making progress. In *bhakti-yoga* one can understand, "Yes, now I am making progress." This is the only *yoga* system by which one can quickly attain self-realization and liberation in this life. One doesn't have to wait for another lifetime.

cañcalaṁ hi manaḥ kṛṣṇa pramāthi balavad dṛḍham
tasyāhaṁ nigrahaṁ manye vāyor iva suduṣkaram

"The mind is restless, turbulent, obstinate, and very strong, O Kṛṣṇa, and to subdue it, I think, is more difficult than controlling the wind." (Bg. 6.34) By chanting Hare Kṛṣṇa, one captures the mind immediately. Just by one's saying the name *Kṛṣṇa* and hearing it, the mind is automatically fixed on Kṛṣṇa. This means that the *yoga* system is immediately attained. The entire *yoga* system aims at concentration on the form of Viṣṇu, and Kṛṣṇa is the original personality from whom all the Viṣṇu forms expand. Kṛṣṇa is like the original candle from which all other candles are lit. If one candle is lit, one can light any number of candles, and there is no doubt that each candle is as powerful as the original candle. Nonetheless, one has to recognize the original candle as the original. Similarly, from Kṛṣṇa millions of Viṣṇu forms expand, and each Viṣṇu form is as good as Kṛṣṇa, but Kṛṣṇa remains the original. Thus one who concentrates his mind on Lord Śrī Kṛṣṇa, the original Supreme Personality of Godhead, immediately attains the perfection of *yoga.*

śrī-bhagavān uvāca
asaṁśayaṁ mahā-bāho mano durnigrahaṁ calam
abhyāsena tu kaunteya vairāgyeṇa ca gṛhyate

"Lord Śrī Kṛṣṇa said: O mighty-armed son of Kuntī, it is undoubtedly very difficult to curb the restless mind, but it is possible by suitable practice and by detachment." (Bg. 6.35) Kṛṣṇa does not say that it is not difficult. Rather, He admits that it is difficult, but He states that it is possible by means of constant practice. Constant practice means engaging ourselves in some activities that remind us of Kṛṣṇa. In the Society for Kṛṣṇa consciousness we therefore have many activities—*kirtana*, temple activities, *prasādam*, publications, and so on. Everyone is engaged in some activity with Kṛṣṇa at the center. Therefore whether one is typing for Kṛṣṇa, cooking for Kṛṣṇa, chanting for Kṛṣṇa, or distributing literature for Kṛṣṇa, he is in the *yoga* system, and he is also in Kṛṣṇa. We engage in activities just as in material life, but these activities are molded in such a way that they are directly connected with Kṛṣṇa. Thus through every activity, Kṛṣṇa consciousness is possible, and perfection in *yoga* follows automatically.

asaṁyatātmanā yogo duṣprāpa iti me matiḥ
vaśyātmanā tu yatatā śakyo 'vāptum upāyataḥ

"For one whose mind is unbridled, self-realization is difficult work. But he whose mind is controlled and who strives by ap-

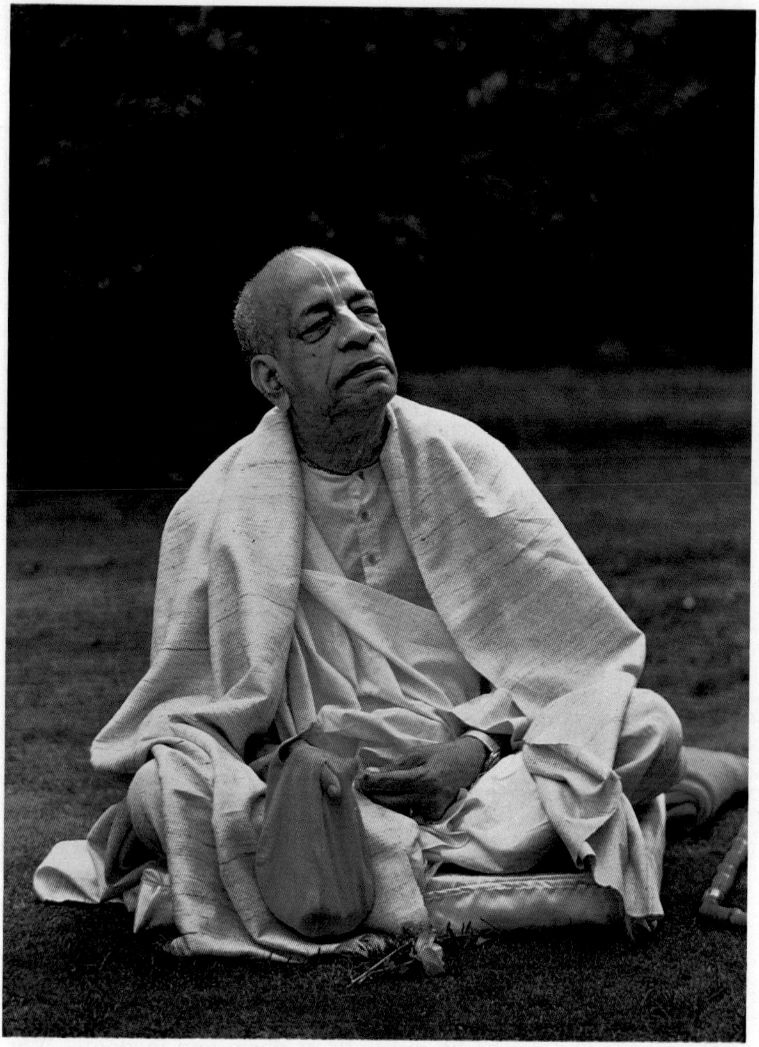

His Divine Grace
A. C. Bhaktivedanta Swami Prabhupāda
Founder-Ācārya of the International Society for Krishna Consciousness
and foremost exponent of yoga in the modern age

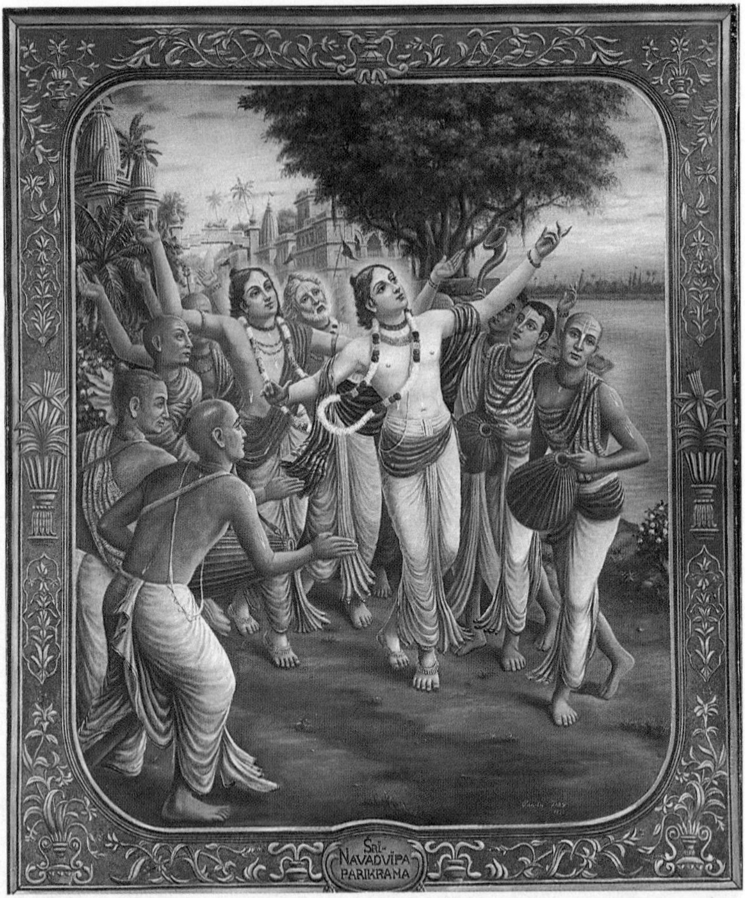

PLATE ONE: Did Caitanya Mahāprabhu sit down to meditate? No, when He propagated *bhakti-yoga* five hundred years ago in India, He was always chanting Hare Kṛṣṇa and dancing. The spirit soul is naturally active. How can we sit down silently and do nothing? It is not possible. No one really wants to sit down and meditate. Why should we? We're meant for positive activity, for recreation, for pleasure. In Kṛṣṇa consciousness, our recreation is dancing and chanting, and when we get tired, we take *prasādam.* Is dancing difficult? Is chanting difficult? It is natural to enjoy music and dancing and palatable foods. These are our recreations, and this is our method of meditation. (*p. 8*)

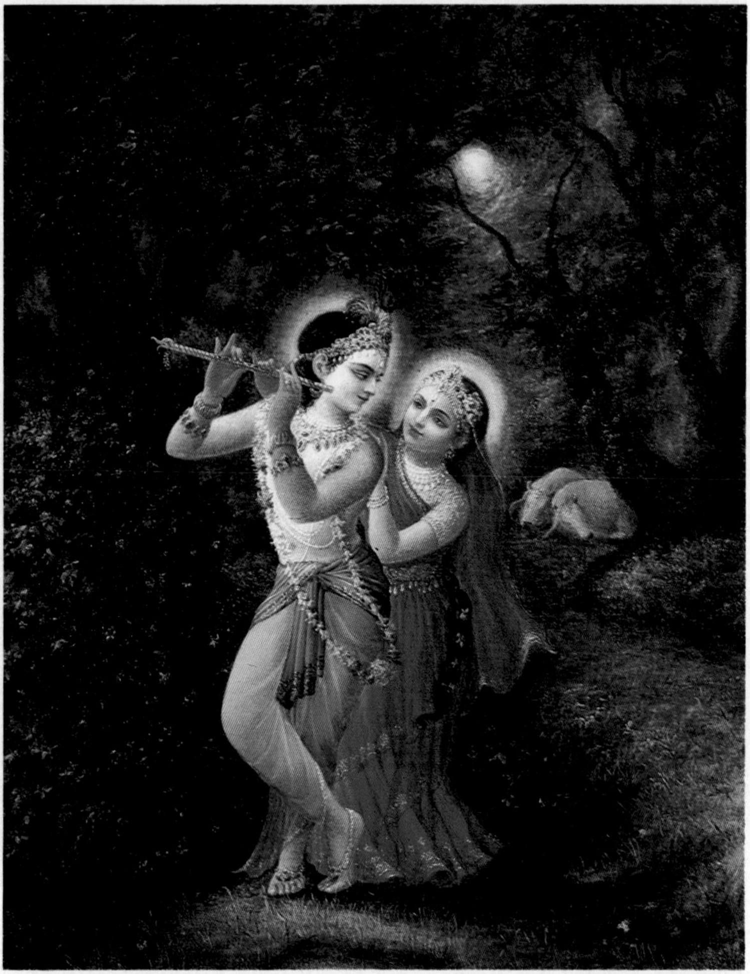

PLATE TWO: The International Society for Krishna Consciousness has been formed to teach people what they have forgotten—the service of Śrī Śrī Rādhā and Kṛṣṇa, the supreme pleasure energy and the Supreme Personality of Godhead. Because we have forgotten the service of Rādhā-Kṛṣṇa, we have become servants of our senses and are experiencing constant frustration. Therefore in this Society we are saying, "You are serving your senses. Now just turn your service to Rādhā and Kṛṣṇa and you will be happy." (*p. 105*)

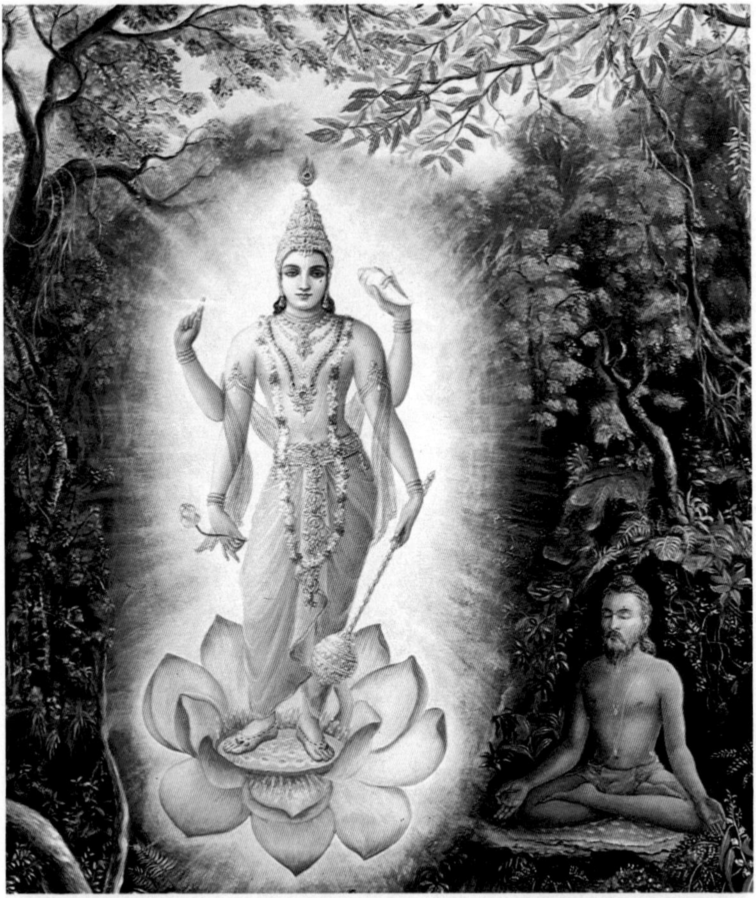

PLATE THREE: One who has developed love for Kṛṣṇa always sees the Lord within his heart. At this stage Lord Kṛṣṇa never disappears from the sight of the devotee, nor does the devotee ever lose sight of the Lord. In the case of a *yogī* who sees the Lord as the Supersoul within the heart, the same applies. Such a *yogī* turns into a pure devotee and cannot bear to live for a moment without seeing the Lord within himself. This is the real process by which we can see God. God is not our order-supplier. We cannot demand, "Come and show Yourself." No, we first have to qualify ourselves. Then we can see God at every moment and everywhere. A *yogī* who is practicing meditation on the Supersoul sees within himself the plenary portion of Kṛṣṇa as Viṣṇu—with four hands, holding conchshell, wheel, club, and lotus flower. (*pp. 77–78*)

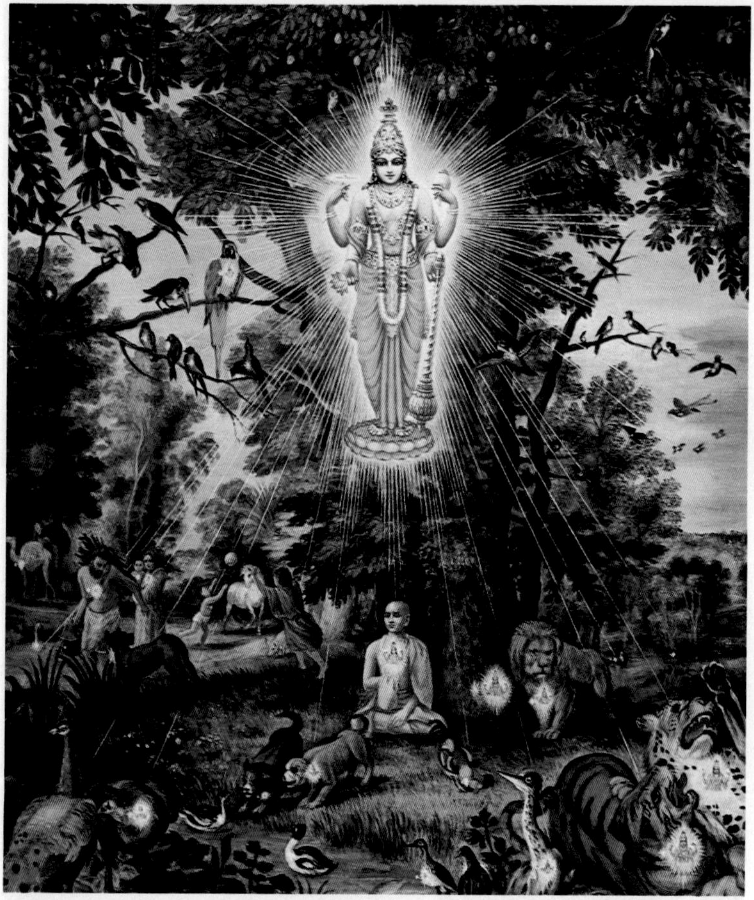

PLATE FOUR: The *yogī* finds out where Lord Viṣṇu is seated within his heart, and when he finds this form there, he concentrates on Him. The *yogī* should know that this Viṣṇu is not different from Kṛṣṇa. Kṛṣṇa in this form of the Supersoul is situated in everyone's heart. Furthermore, there is no difference between the innumerable Supersouls present in the innumerable hearts of the living entities. For example, there is only one sun in the sky, but this sun may be reflected in millions of buckets of water. The sun is one, but it is reflected countless times. According to the *Vedas,* the living entities are innumerable; there is no possibility of counting them. Just as the sun can be reflected in countless buckets of water, Viṣṇu, the Supreme Personality of Godhead, can live in everyone's heart. It is this form upon which the *yogī* concentrates. (*p. 80*)

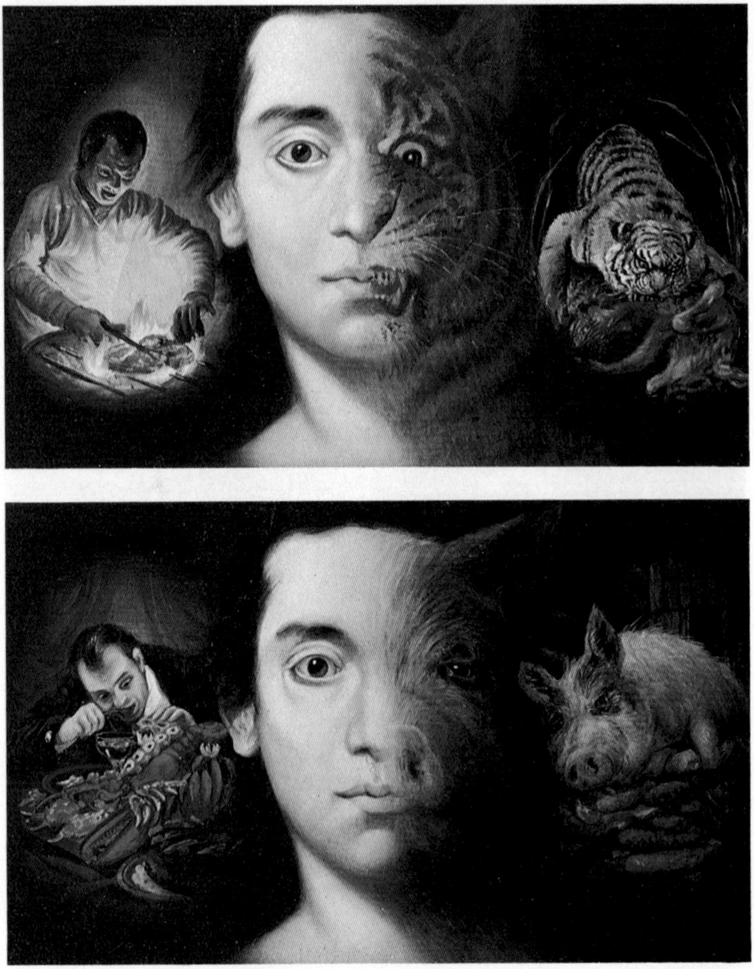

PLATE FIVE: Purification of consciousness is the purpose of *yoga*. At death, the finer elements (mind, intelligence, and ego), which, combined, are called consciousness, carry the small particle of spirit soul to another body to suffer or enjoy according to his work. Different types of bodies are developed according to different types of consciousness. (*p. 93*)

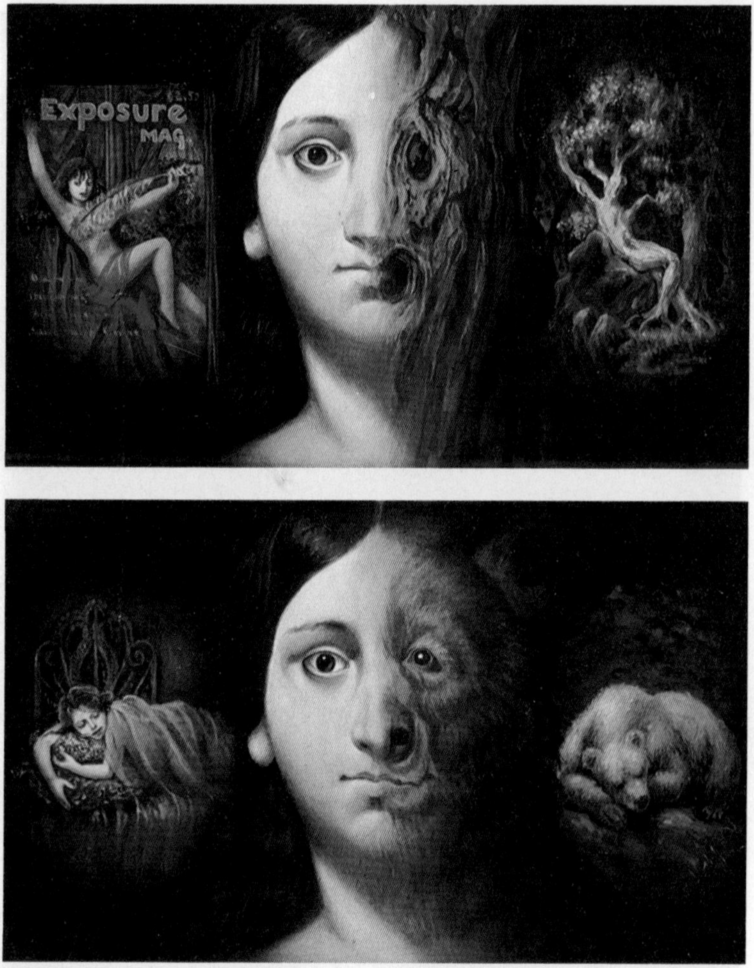

PLATE SIX: One's thoughts and actions in one's present life determine one's consciousness and thus also the type of body one will receive in the next life. A person who likes to eat meat may get a tiger's body, a glutton may get a pig's body, one who likes to expose his or her body may get the body of a tree, which must stand unclothed in all kinds of weather, and one who likes to sleep too much may get a bear's body. (*p. 93*)

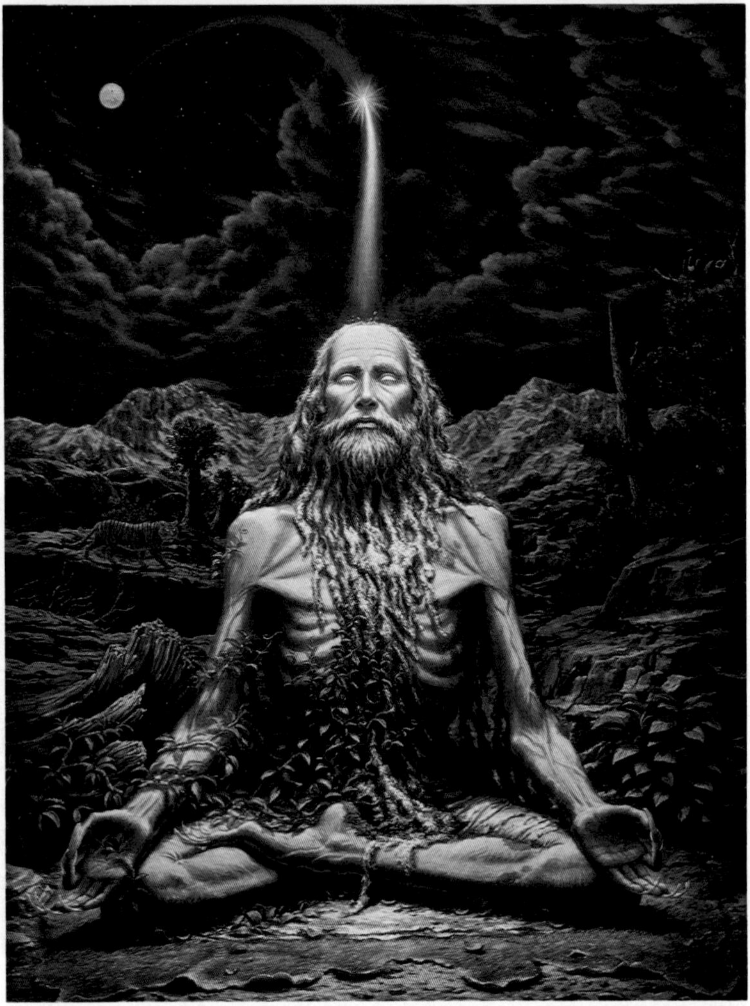

PLATE SEVEN: Genuine *aṣṭāṅga-yogīs* retire to a secluded place for long years of grueling meditation. One of the pitfalls such *yogīs* encounter is subtle material desire. Although Lord Kṛṣṇa declares in the *Bhagavad-gītā* that a *yogī* should be free of all selfish desire, with the advancement of *yoga* one may be tempted by the resultant *siddhis*, or yogic powers, to travel to higher planets or gain some other personal benefit. The *bhakti-yogī* avoids such pitfalls. (*p. 158*)

propriate means is assured of success. That is My opinion." (Bg. 6.36) The Supreme Personality of Godhead declares that one who does not accept the proper treatment to detach the mind from material engagement can hardly achieve success in self-realization. Trying to practice *yoga* while engaging the mind in material enjoyment is like trying to ignite a fire while pouring water on it. Similarly, *yoga* practice without mental control is a waste of time. I may sit down to meditate and focus my mind on Kṛṣṇa, and that is very commendable, but there are many *yoga* societies that teach their students to concentrate on the void or on some color. That is, they do not recommend concentration on the form of Viṣṇu. Trying to concentrate the mind on the impersonal Brahman or the void is very difficult and troublesome. It is stated by Śrī Kṛṣṇa in the Twelfth Chapter of the *Bhagavad-gītā* (12.5),

kleśo 'dhikataras teṣām avyaktāsakta-cetasām
avyaktā hi gatir duḥkhaṁ dehavadbhir avāpyate

"For those whose minds are attached to the unmanifested, impersonal feature of the Supreme, advancement is very troublesome. To make progress in that discipline is always difficult for those who are embodied."

In the temple, the devotee tries to concentrate on the form of Kṛṣṇa. Concentrating on nothingness, on the void, is very difficult, and so naturally, since the mind is very flickering, instead of concentrating on the void the mind searches out something else. The mind must be engaged in thinking of something, and if it is not thinking of Kṛṣṇa, it must be thinking of *māyā*. Therefore, pseudo meditation on the impersonal void is simply a waste of time. Such a show of *yoga* practice may be materially lucrative, but it is useless as far as spiritual realization is concerned. I may open a class in yogic meditation and charge people money for sitting down and pressing their nose this way and that, but if my students do not attain the real goal of *yoga* practice, they have wasted their time and money, and I have cheated them.

Therefore one has to concentrate his mind steadily and constantly on the form of Viṣṇu, and that is called *samādhi*. In Kṛṣṇa consciousness, the mind is controlled by engaging it constantly in the transcendental loving service of the Lord. Unless one is engaged in Kṛṣṇa consciousness, he cannot steadily control the mind. A Kṛṣṇa conscious person easily achieves the result of *yoga* practice without separate endeavor, but a *yoga* practitioner cannot achieve success without becoming Kṛṣṇa conscious.

8
Failure and Success in Yoga

Suppose I give up my business, my ordinary occupation, and begin to practice *yoga*, real *yoga*, as explained herein by Lord Śrī Kṛṣṇa. Suppose I practice, and somehow or other I fail; I cannot properly complete the process. What, then, is the result? This is Arjuna's very next question.

arjuna uvāca
ayatiḥ śraddhayopeto yogāc calita-mānasaḥ
aprāpya yoga-saṁsiddhiṁ kāṁ gatiṁ kṛṣṇa gacchati

"Arjuna said, 'O Kṛṣṇa, what is the destination of the unsuccessful transcendentalist, who in the beginning takes to the process of self-realization with faith but who later desists due to worldly-mindedness and thus does not attain perfection in mysticism?'" (Bg. 6.37)

The path of self-realization, of mysticism, is described in the *Bhagavad-gītā.* The basic principle of self-realization is knowing that "I am not this material body but am different from it, and my happiness is in eternal life, bliss, and knowledge." Before arriving at the point of self-realization, one must take it for granted that he is not the body. That lesson is taught in the very beginning of the *Bhagavad-gītā:* the living entity is not the material body but something different, and his happiness is in eternal life.

Clearly, this life is not eternal. The perfection of *yoga* means attaining a blissful, eternal life full of knowledge. All *yoga* systems should be executed with that goal in mind. It is not that one attends *yoga* classes to reduce fat or to keep the body fit for sense gratification. This is not the goal of *yoga*, but people are taught this way because they want to be cheated. Actually, if you undergo any exercise program, your body will be kept fit. There are many systems of bodily exercise—weightlifting and other sports—and they help keep the body fit, reduce fat, and help the digestive system. Therefore there is no need to practice *yoga* for these purposes. The real purpose of practicing *yoga* is to realize that I am not this body. I want eternal happiness, complete knowledge, and eternal life—that is the ultimate end of the true *yoga* system.

The goal of *yoga* is transcendental, beyond both body and mind. Self-realization is sought by three methods: (1) the path of knowledge (*jñāna*); (2) the path of the eightfold system; or (3) the path of *bhakti-yoga.* In each of these processes, one has to realize the constitutional position of the living entity, his relationship with God, and the activities whereby he can reestablish the lost link and achieve the highest perfectional stage of Kṛṣṇa consciousness. Following any of the above-mentioned three methods, one is sure to reach the supreme goal sooner or later. This was asserted by the Lord in the Second Chapter: even a little endeavor on the transcendental path offers great hope for deliverance.

Of these three methods, the path of *bhakti-yoga* is especially suitable for this age because it is the most direct method of God realization. To be doubly assured, Arjuna is asking Lord Kṛṣṇa to confirm His former statement. One may sincerely accept the path of self-realization, but the process of cultivation of knowledge (*jñāna*) and the practice of the eightfold *yoga* system are generally very difficult for this age. Therefore, despite constant endeavor, one may fail for many reasons. First of all, one may not be actually following the process, the rules and regulations. To pursue the transcendental path is more or less to declare war on the illusory energy. When we accept any process of self-realization, we are actually declaring war against *māyā*, illusion, and *māyā* is certain to place many difficulties before us. So there is a chance of failure, and one has to become very steady. Whenever a person tries to escape the clutches of the illusory energy, she tries to defeat the practitioner by various allurements. A conditioned soul is already allured by the modes of material energy, and there is every chance of being allured again, even while performing transcendental disciplines. This is called *yogāc calita-mānasaḥ,* deviation from the transcendental path. Arjuna is inquisitive to know the results of deviation from the path of self-realization.

As stated in the *Bhagavad-gītā* (6.37), quoted above, *yogāt* means "from the practice of *yoga,*" *calita* means "diversion," and *mānasaḥ* means "mind." So there is every chance for the mind to be diverted from *yoga* practice. We all have some experience of trying to concentrate while reading a book and having our mind be so disturbed that it does not allow us to concentrate on the book.

Actually, Arjuna is asking a very important question, for one is subject to failure in all types of *yoga*—be it the eightfold *yoga* system, the *jñāna-yoga* system of speculative philosophy, or the *bhakti-yoga* system of devotional service. Failure is possible on any of these paths, and the results of failure are clearly explained by Śrī Kṛṣṇa Himself in the following dialogue with Arjuna (Bg. 6.38–44). Arjuna, continuing his inquiry, asks,

kaccin nobhaya-vibhraṣṭaś chinnābhram iva naśyati
apratiṣṭho mahā-bāho vimūḍho brahmaṇaḥ pathi

"O mighty-armed Kṛṣṇa, does not such a man, who is bewildered from the path of transcendence, fall away from both spiritual and material success and perish like a riven cloud, with no position in any sphere?"

etan me saṁśayaṁ kṛṣṇa chettum arhasy aśeṣataḥ
tvad-anyaḥ saṁśayasyāsya chettā na hy upapadyate

"This is my doubt, O Kṛṣṇa, and I ask You to dispel it completely. But for Yourself, no one is to be found who can destroy this doubt."

śrī-bhagavān uvāca
pārtha naiveha nāmutra vināśas tasya vidyate
na hi kalyāṇa-kṛt kaścid durgatiṁ tāta gacchati

"The Supreme Personality of Godhead said, 'O Son of Pṛthā, a transcendentalist engaged in auspicious activities does not meet with destruction either in this world or in the spiritual world; one who does good, My friend, is never overcome by evil.' "

prāpya puṇya-kṛtāṁ lokān uṣitvā śāśvatīḥ samāḥ
śucīnāṁ śrīmatāṁ gehe yoga-bhraṣṭo 'bhijāyate

"The unsuccessful *yogī*, after many, many years of enjoyment on the planets of the pious living entities, is born into a family of righteous people, or into a family of rich aristocracy."

atha vā yoginām eva kule bhavati dhīmatām
etad dhi durlabhataraṁ loke janma yad īdṛśam

"Or he takes his birth in a family of transcendentalists who are surely great in wisdom. Verily, such a birth is rare in this world."

tatra taṁ buddhi-saṁyogaṁ labhate paurva-dehikam
yatate ca tato bhūyaḥ saṁsiddhau kuru-nandana

"On taking such a birth, he revives the divine consciousness of his previous life, and he again tries to make progress in order to achieve complete success, O son of Kuru."

pūrvābhyāsena tenaiva hriyate hy avaśo 'pi saḥ
jijñāsur api yogasya śabda-brahmātivartate

"By virtue of the divine consciousness of his previous life, he automatically becomes attracted to the yogic principles—even without seeking them. Such an inquisitive transcendentalist stands always above the ritualistic principles of the scriptures."

Purification of consciousness is the purpose of the Kṛṣṇa consciousness movement. Presently we are preparing this divine consciousness, for our consciousness goes with us at the time of death. Consciousness is carried from the body just as the aroma of a flower is carried by the air. When we die, the material body composed of five elements—earth, water, fire, air, and ether—decomposes and the gross materials return to the elements. Or, as the Christian Bible says, "Dust thou art, and unto dust thou shalt return." In some societies the body is burned, in others it is buried, and in others it is thrown to animals. In India, the Hindus burn the body, and thus the body is transformed into ashes. Ash is simply another form of earth. Christians bury the body, and after some time in the grave the body eventually turns to dust, which again, like ash, is another form of earth. There are other societies—like the Parsee community in India—that neither burn nor bury the body but throw it to the vultures. The vultures immediately come and eat the body, which is eventually transformed into stool. So in any case, this beautiful body, which we are soaping and caring for so nicely, will eventually turn into either stool, ashes, or dust.

At death, the finer elements (mind, intelligence, and ego), which, combined, are called consciousness, carry the small particle of spirit soul to another body to suffer or enjoy according to his work. Our consciousness is molded by our work. The situation is like what happens when a breeze passes over either a latrine or a rose garden. In one case we say, "Oh, it is a very bad smell," and in the other we say, "It smells very nice." So if we associate with "stool" during our lifetime, our consciousness, which is like the air, will carry the aroma of stool, and thus at the time of death our consciousness will transport us to an undesirable body. Or, if the consciousness passes over "roses," it carries the aroma of roses, and thus we are transported to a body wherein we can enjoy the results of our previous work. And if we train ourselves to work in Kṛṣṇa consciousness, our consciousness will carry us to Kṛṣṇa. Different types of bodies are developed according to different types of consciousness; therefore, if we train our consciousness according to the yogic principles, we will attain a body wherein we can practice *yoga.* We will get good parents and a chance to practice the *yoga* system, and automatically we will be able to revive the Kṛṣṇa consciousness practiced in our previous body. Therefore it is stated in this last verse, "By virtue of the divine consciousness of his previous life, he automatically becomes attracted to the yogic principles—even without seeking them." Therefore, our present duty is to cultivate divine consciousness. If we want divine life, spiritual elevation, and eternal, blissful life, full of knowledge—in other words, if we want to go back home, back to Godhead—we have to train ourselves in divine consciousness, or Kṛṣṇa consciousness.

This can be easily done through association (*saṅgāt sañjāyate kāmaḥ*). Through divine association our consciousness is made divine, and through demoniac association our consciousness is made demoniac. Therefore, our consciousness must be trained to be divine through the proper association of those in Kṛṣṇa consciousness. That is the duty of one in this human form, a form that gives us a chance to make our next life completely divine. To attain this end, we should try to contact those who are developing divine consciousness.

prayatnād yatamānas tu yogī saṁśuddha-kilbiṣaḥ
aneka-janma-saṁsiddhas tato yāti parāṁ gatim

"And when the *yogī* engages himself with sincere endeavor in making further progress, being washed of all contaminations, then ultimately, achieving perfection after many, many births of practice, he attains the supreme goal." (Bg. 6.45) As indicated in this verse, making progress is a question of practice. When a child is born, he knows neither how to smoke nor how to drink, but through association he becomes a smoker and a drunkard. Association is the most important factor. *Saṅgāt sañjāyate kāmaḥ.* For instance, there are many business associations, and by one's becoming a member of certain associations, his business flourishes. In any endeavor, association is very important. For the development of divine consciousness we have established the International Society for Krishna Consciousness, in which the methods of attaining divine consciousness are taught. In this society we invite everyone to come and chant Hare Kṛṣṇa. This process is not difficult, and even children can participate. No previous qualifications are necessary; one doesn't need a master's degree or doctorate. Our invitation to everyone is to join this association and become Kṛṣṇa conscious.

The Supreme Lord, God, is pure, and His kingdom is also pure. If one wants to enter His kingdom, he must also be pure. This is very natural; if we want to enter a particular society, we must meet certain qualifications. If we want to return home, back to Godhead, there is a qualification we must meet—we must not be materially contaminated. And what is this contamination? Unrestricted sense gratification. If we can free ourselves from the material contamination of sense gratification, we can become eligible to enter the kingdom of God. That process of freeing ourselves, of washing ourselves of this contamination, is called the *yoga* system. As stated before, *yoga* does not mean sitting down for fifteen minutes, meditating, and then continuing with sense gratification. To be cured of a certain disease, we must follow the prescriptions of a physician. In the Sixth Chapter of the *Bhagavad-gītā*, the process of *yoga* is recommended, and we have to follow the prescribed methods in order to be freed from material contamination. If we succeed in doing so, we can link up with the Supreme Lord.

Kṛṣṇa consciousness is a method for connecting directly with the Supreme Lord. This is the special gift of Lord Caitanya Mahāprabhu. Not only is this method direct and immediate, but it is also practical. Although many people entering this Society have no qualifications, they have become highly advanced in Kṛṣṇa consciousness simply by coming in contact with the Society. In this age, life is very short, and a *yoga* process that takes a long time will not help the general populace. In Kali-yuga people are also unfortunate, and association is very bad. Therefore, this process of directly contacting the Supreme Lord is recommended—*hari-nāma.* Kṛṣṇa is present in the form of His transcendental name, and we can contact Him immediately by hearing His name. Simply by hearing the name *Kṛṣṇa* we immediately become freed from material contamination.

As stated in the Seventh Chapter of the *Bhagavad-gītā* (7.28),

yeṣāṁ tv anta-gataṁ pāpaṁ janānāṁ puṇya-karmaṇām
te dvandva-moha-nirmuktā bhajante māṁ dṛḍha-vratāḥ

"Persons who have acted piously in previous lives and in this life, whose sinful actions are completely eradicated, and who are freed from the duality of delusion engage themselves in My service with determination." It is herein stressed that one must be completely fixed in Kṛṣṇa consciousness, devoid of duality, and must execute only pious activities. Because the mind is flickering, dualities will always come. One is always wondering, "Shall I become Kṛṣṇa conscious, or should I engage in another consciousness?" These problems are always there, but if one is advanced by virtue of pious activities executed in a previous life, his consciousness will be steadily fixed, and he will resolve, "I will be Kṛṣṇa conscious."

Whether we acted piously in this life or a previous life really doesn't matter. This chanting of Hare Kṛṣṇa is so potent that through it we will immediately be purified. We should have the determination, however, not to become implicated in further impious activities. Therefore, for those who want to be initiated in the Society for Kṛṣṇa consciousness, there are four principles: no illicit sex, no intoxication, no meat-eating, and no gambling. We don't say, "No sex." But we do say, "No illicit sex." If you want sex, get married, and then you can have sex only for having children, not for any other purpose. "No intoxication" means not even taking tea or coffee, to say nothing of other intoxicants. And there is no gambling and no meat-eating (including fish and eggs). Simply by following these four basic rules and regulations, one becomes immediately uncontaminated. No further endeavor is necessary. As soon as one joins the Kṛṣṇa consciousness movement and follows these rules and regulations, material contamination is immediately removed, but one must be careful not to be contaminated again. Therefore these rules and regulations should be followed carefully.

Material contamination begins with these four bad habits, and if we manage to check them, there is no question of contamination. Therefore, as soon as we take to Kṛṣṇa consciousness, we become free. However, we should not think that because Kṛṣṇa consciousness makes us free we can again indulge in these four bad habits and get free by chanting. That is cheating, and that will not be allowed. Once we are freed, we should not allow ourselves to become contaminated again. One should not think, "I shall drink or have illicit sex and then chant and make myself free." According to some religious processes, it is said that one can commit all kinds of sin and then go to church, confess to a priest, and be freed of all sin. Therefore people are sinning and confessing, sinning and confessing, over and over again. But this is not the process of Kṛṣṇa consciousness. If you are freed, that's all right, but don't do it again. After all, what is the purpose of confession? If you confess, "I have committed these sinful activities," why should you commit them again? If a thief confesses that he has been pickpocketing and is freed by virtue of his confession, does this mean he may go out again and freely pick pockets? This requires a little intelligence. One should not think that because by confessing one becomes freed of punishment, he may continue to commit sinful activities, confess again, and again become freed. That is not the purpose of confession.

We should therefore understand that if we indulge in unrestricted sinful activities we become contaminated. We should be careful to have sex only according to the rules and regulations, to eat only food that has been prescribed and properly offered, to defend as Kṛṣṇa advised Arjuna—for the right cause. In this way we can avoid contamination and purify our life. If we can continue to live a pure life until the time of death, we will surely be transferred to the kingdom of God. When one is fully in Kṛṣṇa consciousness, he does not return to this material world when he gives up his body. This is stated in the Fourth Chapter (Bg. 4.9).

janma karma ca me divyam evaṁ yo vetti tattvataḥ
tyaktvā dehaṁ punar janma naiti mām eti so 'rjuna

"One who knows the transcendental nature of My appearance and activities does not, upon leaving the body, take his birth again in this material world, but attains My eternal abode, O Arjuna."

The unsuccessful *yogī* returns to a good family or to a righteous, rich, or aristocratic family, but one who is situated in perfect Kṛṣṇa consciousness does not return. He attains Goloka Vṛndāvana, in the eternal spiritual sky. We should be determined not to come back to this material world, because even if we attain a good birth in a rich or aristocratic family, we can degrade ourselves again by improperly utilizing our good chance. Why take this risk? It is better to complete the process of Kṛṣṇa consciousness in this life. It is very simple and not at all difficult. We only have to keep thinking of Kṛṣṇa; then we will be assured that our next birth will be in the spiritual sky, in Goloka Vṛndāvana, in the kingdom of God.

tapasvibhyo 'dhiko yogī jñānibhyo 'pi mato 'dhikaḥ
karmibhyaś cādhiko yogī tasmād yogī bhavārjuna

"A *yogī* is greater than the ascetic, greater than the empiricist, and greater than the fruitive worker. Therefore, O Arjuna, in all circumstances be a *yogī*." (Bg. 6.46) There are different gradations of life within this material world, but if one lives according to the yogic principles, especially the principles of *bhakti-yoga,* one is living the most perfect life possible. Therefore Kṛṣṇa is telling Arjuna, "My dear friend Arjuna, in all circumstances be a *yogī* and remain a *yogi.*"

yogināṁ api sarveṣāṁ mad-gatenāntarātmanā
śraddhāvān bhajate yo māṁ sa me yuktatamo mataḥ

"And of all *yogīs,* he who always abides in Me with great faith, worshiping Me in transcendental loving service, is most intimately united with Me in *yoga* and is the highest of all." (Bg. 6.47) Here it is clearly stated that there are many types of *yogīs—aṣṭāṅga-yogīs, haṭha-yogīs, jñāna-yogīs, karma-yogīs,* and *bhakti-yogīs*—and that of all the *yogīs,* "he who always abides in Me," is said to be the greatest of all. "In Me" means in Kṛṣṇa; that is, the greatest *yogī* is always in Kṛṣṇa consciousness. Such a *yogī* "abides in Me with great faith, worshiping Me in transcendental loving service, and is thus most intimately united with Me in *yoga* and is the highest of all." This is the prime instruction of this Sixth Chapter on *sāṅkhya-yoga:* if one wants to attain the highest platform of *yoga,* one must remain in Kṛṣṇa consciousness.

In Sanskrit, the word *bhajate,* with its root *bhaj* (*bhaj-dhātu*) means "to render service." But who renders service to Kṛṣṇa unless he is a devotee of Kṛṣṇa? In the Society of Kṛṣṇa consciousness devotees are rendering service without payment, out of love for Kṛṣṇa. They can render service elsewhere and get paid thousands of dollars a month, but the service rendered in the Kṛṣṇa consciousness Society is loving service (*bhaj*)—it is based on love of Godhead. Devotees render service in many ways—gardening, typing, cooking, cleaning, etc. All activities are connected with Kṛṣṇa, and therefore Kṛṣṇa consciousness is prevailing twenty-four hours a day. That is the highest type of *yoga.* That is "worshiping Me in transcendental loving service." As stated before, the perfection of *yoga* is keeping one's consciousness in contact with Viṣṇu, or Kṛṣṇa, the Supreme Lord. We are not simply boasting that even a child can be the highest *yogī* simply by participating in Kṛṣṇa consciousness; no, this is the verdict of authorized scripture—the *Bhagavad-gītā.* These words are not our creation but are specifically stated by Lord Śrī Kṛṣṇa, the Supreme Personality of Godhead Himself.

Actually, worship and service are somewhat different. Worship implies some motive. I worship a friend or an important man because if I can please that person I may derive some profit. Those who worship the demigods worship for some ulterior purpose, and that is condemned in the Seventh Chapter of the *Bhagavad-gītā* (7.20):

kāmais tais tair hṛta-jñānāḥ prapadyante 'nya-devatāḥ
taṁ taṁ niyamam āsthāya prakṛtyā niyatāḥ svayā

"Those whose intelligence has been stolen by material desires surrender unto demigods and follow the particular rules and regulations of worship according to their own natures." Those who are bewildered by lust worship the demigods with a motive; therefore, when we speak of worship, some motive is implied. Service, however, is different, for in service there is no motive. Service is rendered out of love, just as a mother renders service to her child out of love only. Everyone can neglect that child, but the mother cannot, because love is present. Similarly, in devotional service to Kṛṣṇa there is no question of personal motive, for the service is rendered out of pure love. That is the perfection of Kṛṣṇa consciousness.

This is also the recommendation of *Śrīmad-Bhāgavatam* (1.2.6):

sa vai puṁsāṁ paro dharmo yato bhaktir adhokṣaje
ahaituky apratihatā yayātmā suprasīdati

"The supreme occupation [*dharma*] for all humanity is that by which men can attain to loving devotional service unto the transcendent Lord. Such devotional service must be unmotivated and uninterrupted to completely satisfy the self." *Yato bhaktir adhokṣaje.* The word *bhakti* also comes from *bhaj*, the root of the word *bhajate.* The test of a first-class religion is whether or not we are developing our love for God. If we practice religion with some ulterior motive, hoping to fulfill our material necessities, our religion is not first class but third class. It must be understood that first-class religion is that by which we can develop our love of Godhead. *Ahaituky apratihatā.* This perfect religion should be executed without ulterior motive or impediment. That is the *yoga* system recommended in *Śrīmad-Bhāgavatam* and in the Sixth Chapter of the *Bhagavad-gītā*. That is the system of Kṛṣṇa consciousness.

Kṛṣṇa consciousness is not rendered with some material motive in mind. The devotees are not serving Kṛṣṇa in order that He supply them this or that. For a devotee there is no scarcity. One should not think that by becoming Kṛṣṇa conscious one becomes poor. No. If Kṛṣṇa is there, everything is there, because Kṛṣṇa is everything. But this does not mean that we should try to conduct business with Kṛṣṇa, demanding, "Kṛṣṇa, give me this. Give me that." Kṛṣṇa knows what we require better than we do, and He knows our motives. A child does not make demands of his parents, saying, "Dear father, give me this. Give me that." Since the father knows his child's necessities, there is no need for the child to ask. Similarly, it is not a very good idea to ask God to give us this or that. Why should we ask? If God is all-knowing and all-powerful, He knows our necessities and can supply them. This is confirmed in the *Vedas*. *Eko bahūnāṁ yo vidadhāti kāmān:* "The single almighty God is supplying all necessities to millions and trillions of living entities." Therefore, we should not demand anything of God, because our demands are already met. The supplies are already there. We should simply try to love God. Even cats and dogs are receiving their necessities without going to church and petitioning God. If a cat or dog receives its necessities without making demands, why should the devotee not receive what he needs? Therefore we should not demand anything from God but should simply try to love Him. Then everything will be fulfilled, and we will have attained the highest platform of *yoga*.

We can actually see how the various parts of the body serve the body. If I have an itch, the fingers immediately scratch. If I want to see something, the eyes immediately look. If I want to go somewhere, the legs immediately take me. As I receive service from the different parts of my body, God receives service from all parts of His creation. God is not meant to serve. If the limbs of the body serve the entire body, the parts of the body automatically receive energy. Similarly, if we serve Kṛṣṇa, we automatically receive all necessities, all energy.

Śrīmad-Bhāgavatam confirms that we are all parts and parcels of the Supreme. If a part of the body cannot regularly render service, it gives pain to the body, and if a person does not render service to the Supreme Lord, he is simply giving pain and trouble to the Supreme Lord. Therefore such a person has to suffer, just as a criminal has to suffer when he does not abide by the laws of the state. Such a criminal may think, "I'm a very good man," but because he is violating the laws of the state, he is giving the government trouble, and consequently the government puts him in prison. When living entities give the Supreme Lord trouble, the Lord comes, collects them together, and puts them in this material world. In essence, He says, "You live here. You are all disturbing the creation; therefore you are criminals and have to live in this material world." *Sthānād bhraṣṭāḥ patanty adhaḥ:* "One falls down from his constitutional position." If a finger is diseased, it has to be amputated lest it pollute the entire body. Having rebelled against the principles of God consciousness, we are cut off from our original position. We have fallen. In order to regain our original position, we must resume rendering service unto the Supreme Lord. That is the perfect cure. Otherwise we will continue to suffer pain, and God will suffer pain because of us. If I am a father and my son is not good, I suffer and my son suffers also. Similarly, we are all sons of God, and when we cause God pain we are also pained. The best course is to revive our original Kṛṣṇa consciousness and engage in the Lord's service. That is our natural life, and that is possible in the spiritual sky, Goloka Vṛndāvana.

The word *avajānanti* actually means "to neglect." This means thinking, "What is God? I am God. Why should I serve God?" This is just like a criminal thinking, "What is this government? I can manage my own affairs. I don't care for the government." This is called *avajānanti.* We may speak in this way, but the police department is there to punish us. Similarly, material nature is here to punish us with the threefold miseries. These miseries are meant for those rascals who don't care for God or who take the meaning of *God* cheaply, saying, "I am God. You are God."

Thus the general progress of *yoga* is gradual. First one practices *karma-yoga*, which refers to ordinary, fruitive activity. Ordinary activities include sinful activities, but *karma-yoga* excludes such activities. *Karma-yoga* refers only to good, pious activities, or those actions which are prescribed. After performing *karma-yoga*, one comes to the platform of *jñāna-yoga*, knowledge. From the platform of knowledge, one attains to this *aṣṭāṅga-yoga*, the eightfold *yoga* system—*āsana, prāṇāyāma, dhāraṇā, dhyāna,* etc.—and from *aṣṭāṅga-yoga,* as one concentrates on Viṣṇu, one comes to the point of *bhakti-yoga. Bhakti-yoga* is the perfectional stage, and if one practices Kṛṣṇa consciousness, one attains this stage from the very beginning. That is the direct route.

If one practices *jñāna-yoga* and thinks that he has attained the ultimate, he is mistaken. He has to make further progress. If we are on a staircase and want to reach the top floor, which is the hundredth floor, we are mistaken if we think we have arrived when we are on the thirtieth floor. As stated before, the whole *yoga* system may be likened to a staircase linking us to God. In order to attain the ultimate, the Supreme Personality of Godhead, we must go to the highest platform, and that is *bhakti-yoga.*

But why walk up all these steps if we have a chance to take an elevator? By means of an elevator, we can reach the top in a matter of seconds. *Bhakti-yoga* is this elevator, the direct process by which we can reach the top in a matter of seconds. We can go step by step, following all the other *yoga* systems, or we can go directly. Since in this Age of Kali people have short life spans and are always disturbed and anxious, Lord Caitanya Mahāprabhu, by His causeless mercy, has given us the elevator by which we can come immediately to the platform of *bhakti-yoga.* That direct means is the chanting of Hare Kṛṣṇa, and that is the special gift of Lord Caitanya Mahāprabhu. Therefore Rūpa Gosvāmī offers respects to Lord Caitanya Mahāprabhu, *namo mahā-vadānyāya kṛṣṇa-prema-pradāya te:* "Oh, You are the most munificent incarnation because You are directly giving love of Kṛṣṇa. To attain pure love of Kṛṣṇa one has to pass through so many stages of *yoga,* but You are giving this love directly. Therefore You are the most munificent."

As Kṛṣṇa states in the Eighteenth Chapter of the *Bhagavad-gītā* (18.55),

> *bhaktyā mām abhijānāti yāvān yaś cāsmi tattvataḥ*
> *tato māṁ tattvato jñātvā viśate tad-anantaram*

"One can understand Me as I am, as the Supreme Personality of Godhead, only by devotional service. And when one is in full consciousness of Me by such devotion, he can enter into the kingdom of God." In the other *yoga* systems, there must be a mixture of *bhakti* for one to achieve any success, but *bhakti-yoga* is unadulterated devotion. It is service without a material motive. Generally people pray with some material motive in mind, but we should pray only for further engagement in devotional service. Lord Caitanya Mahāprabhu has taught us that when we pray we should not pray for anything material. In the beginning, we cited Lord Caitanya Mahāprabhu's perfect prayer:

na dhanaṁ na janaṁ na sundarīṁ
kavitāṁ vā jagad-īśa kāmaye
mama janmani janmanīśvare
bhavatād bhaktir ahaitukī tvayi

"O Almighty Lord, I have no desire to accumulate wealth, nor to enjoy beautiful women. Nor do I want any number of followers. I only want the causeless mercy of Your devotional service in My life, birth after birth." (*Śikṣāṣṭaka* 4) In this verse Caitanya Mahāprabhu addresses the Supreme Lord as Jagadīśa. *Jagat* means "universe," and *īśa* means "controller." The Supreme Lord is the controller of the universe, and this can be understood by anyone; therefore Caitanya Mahāprabhu addresses the Supreme Lord as Jagadīśa instead of Kṛṣṇa or Rāma. In the material world we find many controllers, so it is logical that there is a controller of the entire universe. Caitanya Mahāprabhu does not pray for wealth, followers, or beautiful women, because these are material requests. Usually, people want to be very great leaders within this material world. Someone tries to become a very rich man like Ford or Rockefeller, or someone else tries to become president or some great leader that many thousands of people will follow. These are all material demands: "Give me money. Give me followers. Give me a nice wife." Lord Caitanya Mahāprabhu refuses to make such materialistic requests. He frankly says, "I don't want any of these things." He even says, *mama janmani janmanīśvare.* That is, He's not even asking for liberation. Just as the materialists have their demands, the *yogīs* demand liberation. But Caitanya Mahāprabhu does not want anything of this nature. Then why is He a devotee? Why is He worshiping Kṛṣṇa? "I simply want to engage in Your service birth after birth." He does not even pray for an end to birth, old age, disease, and death. There are no material demands whatsoever. This is the highest platform, the stage of pure *bhakti-yoga.*

When we chant Hare Kṛṣṇa we are also asking the Lord, "Please engage me in Your service." This is the *mantra* taught by Caitanya Mahāprabhu Himself. *Hare* refers to the energy of the Lord, and *Kṛṣṇa* and *Rāma* are names for the Lord Himself. When we chant Hare Kṛṣṇa, we are asking Kṛṣṇa to please engage us in His service. This is because our entire material disease is due to our having forgotten to serve God. In illusion, we are thinking, "I am God. What is some other God that I have to serve? I myself am God." Ultimately, that is the only disease, the last snare of illusion. First of all, a person tries to be prime minister, president, Rockefeller, Ford, this and that, and when one fails to become happy in this way, he wants to become God. That is like becoming an even higher president. When I understand that the presidency does not afford me eternal bliss and knowledge, I demand the highest presidency. I demand to become God. In any case, the demand is there, and this demand is our disease. In illusion, we are demanding to be the highest, but the process of *bhakti-yoga* is just the opposite. We want to become servants, servants of the servants of the Lord. There is no question of demanding to become the Lord; we just want to serve. That's all.

Our original nature is rooted in service, and wanting to serve is the crucial test for the devotee. We may not realize it, but in this material world we are also serving. If we want to become president, we have to make so many promises to the voters. In other words, the president has to say, "I'll give the people my service." Unless he promises to serve his country, there is no question of his becoming president. So even if one is the most exalted leader, his position is to render service. This is very difficult for people to understand. Despite becoming the highest executive in the land, one has to give service to the people. If that service is not given, one is likely to be usurped, fired, or killed. In the material world, service is very dangerous. If there is a little discrepancy in one's service, one is immediately fired. When the people did not like the service that President Nixon was rendering, they forced him to resign. Some people disagreed with President Kennedy, and he was killed. Similarly, in India, Mahatma Gandhi was also killed because some people did not like the way he was rendering service. This is always the position in the material world; therefore one should be intelligent enough to decide to cease rendering service for material motives. We must render service to the Supreme Lord, and that rendering of service is our perfection.

We have formed the International Society for Krishna Consciousness in order to teach people what they have forgotten. In this material world, we have forgotten the service of Rādhā-Kṛṣṇa; therefore we have become servants of *māyā,* the senses. Therefore, in this Society we are saying, "You are serving your senses. Now just turn your service to Rādhā and Kṛṣṇa, and you will be happy. You have to render service—either to *māyā* [illusion] and your senses, or to Śrī Śrī Rādhā-Kṛṣṇa."

In this world, everyone is serving the senses, but people are not satisfied. No one can be satisfied, because the senses are always demanding more gratification, and this means that we are constantly having to serve the senses. In any case, our position as servant remains the same. It is a question of whether we want to be happy in our service. It is the verdict of the *Bhagavad-gītā* and the other Vedic scriptures that we will never be happy trying to serve our senses, for they are only sources of misery. Therefore Lord Caitanya Mahāprabhu prays to be situated in Kṛṣṇa's service. He also prays,

ayi nanda-tanuja kiṅkaraṁ
patitaṁ māṁ viṣame bhavāmbudhau
kṛpayā tava pāda-paṅkaja-
sthita-dhūlī-sadṛśaṁ vicintaya

"O son of Mahārāja Nanda [Kṛṣṇa], I am Your eternal servitor, yet somehow or other I have fallen into the ocean of birth and death. Please pick Me up from this ocean of death and place Me as one of the atoms at Your lotus feet." (*Śikṣāṣṭaka* 5) This is another way of asking Kṛṣṇa to engage us in His service.

Loving devotional service can only be rendered to the personal form of Kṛṣṇa, Śyāmasundara. The impersonalists emphasize the *virāṭ-rūpa,* the universal form exhibited in the Eleventh Chapter of the *Bhagavad-gītā,* but it is stated therein

(11.21) that the demigods are very much afraid of this form, and Arjuna says,

adṛṣṭa-pūrvaṁ hṛṣito 'smi dṛṣṭvā
bhayena ca pravyathitaṁ mano me
tad eva me darśaya deva rūpaṁ
prasīda deveśa jagan-nivāsa

"After seeing this universal form, which I have never seen before, I am gladdened, but at the same time my mind is disturbed with fear. Therefore please bestow Your grace upon me and reveal again Your form as the Personality of Godhead [Kṛṣṇa, or Śyāmasundara], O Lord of lords, O abode of the universe." (Bg. 11.45) There is no question of loving the *virāṭ-rūpa.* If Kṛṣṇa comes before you in the *virāṭ-rūpa* form, you will be so filled with fear that you will forget your love. So don't be eager like the impersonalists to see the *virāṭ-rūpa* form; just render loving service to Śyāmasundara, Kṛṣṇa.

We have more or less seen Kṛṣṇa as the *viśva-rūpa* during wartime in Calcutta in 1942. There was a siren, and we ran into a shelter, and the bombing began. In this way, we were seeing that *viśva-rūpa*, and I was thinking, "Of course, this is also just another form of Kṛṣṇa. But this is not a very lovable form." A devotee wants to love Kṛṣṇa in His original form, and this *viśva-rūpa* is not His original form. Being omnipotent, Kṛṣṇa can appear in any form, but His lovable form is that of Kṛṣṇa, Śyāmasundara. Although a man may be a police officer, when he is at home he is a beloved father to his son. But if he comes home firing his revolver, the son will be so frightened that he will forget that he is his beloved father. Naturally, the child loves his father when he's at home like a father, and similarly we love Kṛṣṇa as He is in His eternal abode, in the form of Śyāmasundara.

The *viśva-rūpa* was shown to Arjuna to warn those rascals who claim, "I am God." Arjuna asked to see the *viśva-rūpa* so that in the future we may have some criterion by which to test rascals who claim to be God. In other words, if someone says, "I am God," we can simply reply, "If you are God, please show me your *viśva-rūpa.*" And we can rest assured that such rascals cannot display this form.

Of course, Arjuna was offering all respects to the *viśva-rūpa* form. That is a natural quality of a devotee. A devotee even respects Durgā, Māyā, because Māyā is Kṛṣṇa's energy. If we respect Kṛṣṇa, we respect everyone, even an ant. Therefore Brahmā prays,

sṛṣṭi-sthiti-pralaya-sādhana-śaktir ekā
chāyeva yasya bhuvanāni bibharti durgā
icchānurūpam api yasya ca ceṣṭate sā
govindam ādi-puruṣaṁ tam ahaṁ bhajāmi

"The external potency, Māyā, who is of the nature of the shadow of the *cit* [spiritual] potency, is worshiped by all people as Durgā, the creating, preserving, and destroying agency of this mundane world. I worship the primeval Lord, Govinda, in accordance with whose will Durgā conducts herself." (*Brahma-saṁhitā* 5.44) Thus when we pray to Kṛṣṇa, we pray to Durgā immediately, because Durgā is His energy. And when we pray to Durgā, we are actually praying to Kṛṣṇa, because she is working under the direction of Kṛṣṇa. When the devotee sees the activities of Māyā, he sees Kṛṣṇa immediately, thinking, "Oh, Māyā is acting so nicely under the direction of Kṛṣṇa." When one offers respect to a policeman, he is actually offering respect to the government. Durgā, the material energy, is so powerful that she can create, annihilate, and maintain, but in all cases she is acting under Kṛṣṇa's directions.

Through *bhakti,* pure devotion to Kṛṣṇa, we can leave the association of Māyā and be promoted to the eternal association of Kṛṣṇa. Some of the *gopas,* Kṛṣṇa's friends, are eternal associates, and others are promoted to that eternal position. If only the eternal associates of Kṛṣṇa can play with Him and others cannot, then what is the meaning of becoming Kṛṣṇa conscious? We can also become eternal associates of Kṛṣṇa through pious deeds executed in many, many lives. Actually, in the Vṛndāvana manifest in this material world, the associates of Kṛṣṇa are mainly conditioned living entities who have been promoted to the perfect stage of Kṛṣṇa consciousness. Thus promoted, they are first of all allowed to see Kṛṣṇa on the planet where Kṛṣṇa's pastimes are being enacted. After this, they are promoted to the transcendental Goloka Vṛndāvana in the spiritual sky. Therefore it is stated in the *Bhāgavata* (10.12.11), *kṛta-puṇya-puñjāḥ.*

Bhakti-yoga means connecting ourselves with Kṛṣṇa, God, and becoming His eternal associates. *Bhakti-yoga* cannot be applied to any other objective; therefore in Buddhism, for instance, there is no *bhakti-yoga,* because they do not recognize the Supreme Lord as the supreme objective. Christians, however, practice *bhakti-yoga* when they worship Jesus Christ, because they are accepting him as the son of God and are therefore accepting God. Unless one accepts God, there is no question of *bhakti-yoga.* Christianity, therefore, is also a form of Vaiṣṇavism, because God is recognized. Nonetheless, there are different stages of God realization. Mainly, Christianity says, "God is great," and that is a very good assertion, but the actual greatness of God can be understood from the *Bhagavad-gītā* and *Śrīmad-Bhāgavatam.* Accepting the greatness of God is the beginning of *bhakti. Bhakti-yoga* also exists among the Muslims, because God is the target in the Muslim religion. However, where there is no recognition of a personal God—in other words, where there is only impersonalism—there is no question of *bhakti-yoga. Bhakti-yoga* must include three items: the servitor, the served, and service. Someone must be present to accept service, and someone must be present to render service. The via medium is the process of service itself, *bhakti-yoga.* Now, if there is no one to accept that service, how is *bhakti-yoga* possible? Therefore, if a philosophy or religion does not accept God as the Supreme Person, there is no possibility of *bhakti-yoga* being applied.

In the *bhakti-yoga* process, the role of the spiritual master is most important and essential. Although the spiritual master will always come back until his devotees have achieved God realization, one should not try to take advantage of this. We should not trouble our spiritual master but should complete the *bhakti-yoga* process in this life. The disciple should be serious in his service to the spiritual master, and if the devotee is intelligent, he should think, "Why should I act in such a way that my spiritual master has to take the trouble to reclaim me again? Let me realize Kṛṣṇa in this life." That is the proper way of thinking. We should not think, "Oh, I am sure that my spiritual master will come and save me. Therefore I will do as

I please." If we have any affection for our spiritual master, we should complete the process in this life so that he does not have to return to reclaim us.

In this regard, there is the example of Bilvamaṅgala Ṭhākura, who in his previous life was elevated almost to *prema-bhakti*, the highest platform of devotional service. However, since there is always a chance of a falldown, somehow or other he fell down. In his next life he was born in a very rich *brāhmaṇa* family, in accordance with the principle enunciated in the Sixth Chapter of the *Bhagavad-gītā* (6.41): *śucīnāṁ śrīmatāṁ gehe.* Unfortunately, as is often the case with rich boys, he became a prostitute hunter. Yet it is said that his spiritual master instructed him through his prostitute, saying, "Oh, you are so attached to this mere flesh and bones. If you were this much attached to Kṛṣṇa, how much good you might achieve!" Immediately Bilvamaṅgala Ṭhākura resumed his devotional service.

Although the spiritual master assumes responsibility for his disciple, we should not take advantage of this. Rather, we should try to please the spiritual master (*yasya prasādād bhagavat-prasādaḥ*). We should not put our spiritual master in such a position that he has to reclaim us from a house of prostitution. But even if he has to do so, he will do it, because he assumes this responsibility when he accepts his disciple.

The *bhakti-yoga* process should be completed in this life, because in this life we have all the instruments necessary to become fully Kṛṣṇa conscious. We have tongues with which to chant Hare Kṛṣṇa, and we have ears to hear the sound that the tongue vibrates. Therefore we have all the instruments we need with us—a tongue and ears. We have only to chant Hare Kṛṣṇa and use our ears to hear this vibration, and all perfection will be there. We don't have to become highly educated scientists or philosophers. We have only to chant and hear.

Thus we have everything complete. *Pūrṇam adaḥ pūrṇam idam:* everything created by God is complete. This aggregate earth, for instance, is complete. There is sufficient water in the oceans, and the sun acts to evaporate this water, turn it into clouds, and drop rain on the land to produce plants. And from the mountains, pure rivers are flowing to supply water throughout the year. If we want to evaporate a few hundred gallons of water, we have to make many arrangements, but the creation is so complete that millions of tons of water are being drawn from the ocean, turned into clouds, and then sprayed all over the land and reserved on the peaks of mountains so that water will be present for the production of grains and vegetables. Thus the creation is complete because it comes from the complete, and similarly our bodies are also complete for spiritual realization. The complete machine is already with us. We have only to utilize it to vibrate the transcendental sound (*śabda*) of Hare Kṛṣṇa, and we will attain complete liberation from all material pangs.

9

Destination after Death

sarva-dvārāṇi saṁyamya mano hṛdi nirudhya ca
mūrdhny ādhāyātmanaḥ prāṇam āsthito yoga-dhāraṇām

"The yogic situation is that of detachment from all sensual engagements. Closing all the doors of the senses and fixing the mind on the heart and the life air at the top of the head, one establishes himself in *yoga.*" (Bg. 8.12)

One translation of the word *yoga* is "plus"—that is, just the opposite of minus. At the present moment, due to our materially contaminated consciousness, we are minus God. When we add God to our lives, when we connect with Him, life is perfected. This process has to be finished at the time of death; therefore as long as we are alive, we have to practice approaching that point of perfection so that at the time of death, when we give up this material body, we can realize the Supreme.

prayāṇa-kāle manasācalena
bhaktyā yukto yoga-balena caiva
bhruvor madhye prāṇam āveśya samyak
sa taṁ paraṁ puruṣam upaiti divyam

"One who, at the time of death, fixes his life air between the eyebrows and, by the strength of *yoga*, with an undeviating mind, engages himself in remembering the Supreme Lord in full devotion, will certainly attain to the Supreme Personality of Godhead." (Bg. 8.10) The words *prayāṇa-kāle* mean "at the time of death." Life is kind of a preparation for the final examination, which is death. If we pass that examination, we are transferred to the spiritual world. According to a very common Bengali proverb, "Whatever you do for perfection will be tested at the time of your death."

This process by which the *yogī* closes the doors of the senses is technically called *pratyāhāra,* meaning "just the opposite of sense gratification." Presently, our senses are engaged in seeing worldly beauty. So *pratyāhāra* means retracting the senses from that beauty and seeing the beauty inside. Hearing is concentrated on the *oṁkāra* sound that is within. Similarly, all the other senses are withdrawn from external activity. The mind is then concentrated on the form of Lord Viṣṇu within the heart (*manaḥ hṛdi nirudhya*). The word *nirudhya* means "confining" the mind within the heart. When the *yogī* has thus withdrawn his senses and concentrated his mind, he transfers the life air to the top of the head and decides where he should go. There are innumerable planets, and beyond these planets is the spiritual world. The *yogīs* obtain information of these planets from the Vedic literatures, just as, before coming to the United States, I obtained information about this country from books. Since all the higher planets in the spiritual world are described in the Vedic literatures, the *yogī* knows everything and can transfer himself to any planet he likes. He does not need a material spaceship.

Scientists have been trying for many years to reach other planets with spaceships, but this is not the process. Maybe by this means one or two men can reach a planet, but that is not the general process. It is not possible for everyone. Generally, if one wants to transfer himself to a higher planet, he practices this *jñāna-yoga* system. Not the *bhakti-yoga* system. The system of *bhakti-yoga* is not used for attaining any material planet.

The devotees of Kṛṣṇa are not interested in any planet within this material universe, because they know that on all planets the four basic miseries exist—birth, old age, disease, and death. In the higher planets, one's life span may be much greater than on this earth, but death is ultimately there. Therefore those who are in Kṛṣṇa consciousness are interested not in material life but in spiritual life, which means relief from these fourfold miseries. Those who are intelligent do not try to elevate themselves to any planet within this material world. To attain a higher planet, one has to prepare a particular type of body to enable one to live on that planet. We cannot attain these planets by artificial, materialistic means, because a suitable body is necessary to live there. We can stay within water only a short while, but fish are living there their entire lives. But the fish do not have bodies suitable for living on the land. Similarly, to enter a higher planet, one has to acquire a suitable body.

In the higher planets, one day and night is equal to one of our years, and the inhabitants of these planets live ten thousand celestial years. This is all described in the Vedic literatures. Although the life span on these planets is very long, there is ultimately death. After ten thousand years, twenty thousand years, or millions of years—it doesn't matter—death is ultimately there.

In the very beginning of the *Bhagavad-gītā*, however, we learn that we are not subject to death.

na jāyate mriyate vā kadācin
nāyaṁ bhūtvā bhavitā vā na bhūyaḥ
ajo nityaḥ śāśvato 'yaṁ purāṇo
na hanyate hanyamāne śarīre

"For the soul there is neither birth nor death at any time. He has not come into being, does not come into being, and will not come into being. He is unborn, eternal, ever-existing and primeval. He is not slain when the body is slain." (Bg. 2.20) Kṛṣṇa thus instructs us that we are spirit soul and eternal; therefore why should we subject ourselves to birth and death? One who utilizes his intelligence can understand this. One who is situated in Kṛṣṇa consciousness is not interested in promotion to any planet where death exists; rather, being promoted to the spiritual sky, he receives a body just like God's. *Īśvaraḥ paramaḥ kṛṣṇaḥ sac-cid-ānanda-vigrahaḥ.* God's body is *sac-cid-ānanda*—eternal, full of knowledge, and full of pleasure. Therefore Kṛṣṇa is called the reservoir of all pleasure. If, upon leaving this body, we transfer ourselves to the spiritual world—to Kṛṣṇa's planet or any other spiritual planet—we attain a similar *sac-cid-ānanda* body.

The spirit soul is a very minute particle within the body. It cannot be seen like the external body, but it is sustaining the external body. The object of the system of meditative *yoga* (*aṣṭāṅga-yoga* or *dhyāna-yoga*) is to bring the soul to the topmost part of the head. From there, one who is perfect in *dhyāna-yoga* can transfer himself to a higher planet at will. That is the perfection of this type of *yoga.* The *dhyāna-yogī* is somewhat like a traveler who thinks, "Oh, let me see what the moon is like; then I will transfer myself to higher planets." He goes from here to there in the universe, just as on earth travelers go from New York to California or Canada. But a Kṛṣṇa conscious person is not interested in such interplanetary travel within the material universe. His goal is service to Kṛṣṇa and transferal to the spiritual sky.

oṁ ity ekākṣaraṁ brahma vyāharan mām anusmaran
yaḥ prayāti tyajan dehaṁ sa yāti paramāṁ gatim

"After being situated in this *yoga* practice and vibrating the sacred syllable *oṁ*, the supreme combination of letters, if one thinks of the Supreme Personality of Godhead and quits his body, he will certainly reach the spiritual planets." (Bg. 8.13) *Oṁ*, or *oṁkāra*, is the concise form of the transcendental vibration. The *dhyāna-yogī* should vibrate *oṁ* while remembering Kṛṣṇa, or Viṣṇu, the Supreme Personality of Godhead. The impersonal sound of Kṛṣṇa is *oṁ*, but the sound *Hare Kṛṣṇa* contains *oṁ*. Whatever the case, the entire *yoga* system aims at concentration on Viṣṇu. Impersonalists may imagine a form of Viṣṇu, but the personalists do not imagine; they actually *see* the form of the Supreme Lord. Whether one imagines or factually sees, one has to concentrate his mind on the Viṣṇu form. Here the word *mām* means "unto the Supreme Lord, Viṣṇu." If one can remember Viṣṇu upon quitting this body, he can enter into the spiritual kingdom.

One who is intelligent naturally thinks, "I am permanent and eternal. Why should I be interested in things that are not permanent?" Actually, no one wants an existence that is temporary. If we are living in an apartment and the landlord asks us to vacate, we have to do so, whether we want to leave or not. However, if we move to a better apartment, we are not sorry. It is our nature, however, to want to remain wherever we live. That is because we are permanent and want a permanent residence. Our inclination is to remain. Therefore we don't want to die. We don't want the miseries of birth, old age, disease, and death. These are external miseries inflicted by material nature, and they attack us like some fever. In order to extricate ourselves, we have to take certain precautions. To get rid of these miseries, it is necessary to get rid of the material body, because these miseries are inherent in material existence.

Thus by vibrating *oṁ* and leaving the material body thinking of the Supreme Lord, the *yogī* is transferred to the spiritual world. Those who are not personalists, however, cannot enter into the spiritual planet of Lord Śrī Kṛṣṇa. They remain outside, in the *brahmajyoti* effulgence. Just as the sunshine is not different from the sun globe, the *brahmajyoti* effulgence of the Supreme Lord is not different from the Supreme Lord. The impersonalists are placed in that *brahmajyoti* as minute particles. We are all spiritual sparks, and the *brahmajyoti* is full of these spiritual sparks. In this way, the impersonalists merge into the spiritual existence; however, individuality is retained, because the spirit soul is constitutionally an individual. Because the impersonalists don't want a personal form, they are placed into the impersonal *brahmajyoti* and held there, where they exist just as atoms exist within the sunshine. The individual spiritual spark remains within the *brahmajyoti* as if homogeneous.

As living entities, we all want enjoyment. We do not simply want existence. We are constitutionally *sac-cid-ānanda*—eternal (*sat*), full of knowledge (*cit*), and full of bliss (*ānanda*). Those who enter the impersonal *brahmajyoti* cannot remain there eternally with the knowledge that "Now I am merged. I am now one with Brahman." Although there is eternality and knowledge, bliss (*ānanda*) is lacking. Who can remain alone in a room year after year reading some book and trying to enjoy himself? We cannot remain alone forever. Eventually we will leave that room and look for some association. It is our nature to want some recreation with others. Therefore the impersonalists, dissatisfied with the loneliness of their position in the impersonal effulgence of the Lord, return again to this material world. This is stated in *Śrīmad-Bhāgavatam* (10.2.32):

ye 'nye 'ravindākṣa vimukta-māninas
tvayy asta-bhāvād aviśuddha-buddhayaḥ
āruhya kṛcchreṇa paraṁ padaṁ tataḥ
patanty adho 'nādṛta-yuṣmad-aṅghrayaḥ

"O lotus-eyed Lord, although nondevotees who accept severe austerities and penances to achieve the highest position may think themselves liberated, their intelligence is impure. They fall down from their position of imagined superiority because they have no regard for Your lotus feet."

The impersonalists are like astronauts in search of a planet. If they cannot rest on some planet, they have to return to earth. It is herein stated in *Śrīmad-Bhāgavatam* (*anādṛta-yuṣmad-aṅghrayaḥ*) that the impersonalist must return to the material world because he has neglected to serve the Supreme Lord with love and devotion. As long as we are on this earth, we should practice to love and serve Kṛṣṇa, the Supreme Lord; then we can enter His spiritual planet. If we are not trained up in this way, we can enter the *brahmajyoti* as an impersonalist, but there is every risk that we will again fall down into material existence. Out of loneliness, we will search out some association and therefore return to the material world. What we actually want is the eternal association of the Supreme Lord. This is our constitutional position of eternality, knowledge, and pleasure. If we are alone, if we do not associate with the Supreme Lord, that pleasure is lacking. For want of pleasure, we feel uncomfortable. For want of pleasure, we will accept any kind of association, any kind of pleasure. Therefore, out of a kind of desperation, we will say, "All right, then let me have material pleasure again." That is the risk the impersonalists take.

In the material world, the highest pleasure is found in sex. That is but a perverted reflection of the pleasure experienced with Kṛṣṇa in the spiritual world. Unless there is sex in the spiritual world, it cannot be reflected here. However, we should understand that here the reflection is perverted. Actual life is there in Kṛṣṇa. Kṛṣṇa is full of pleasure, and if we train ourselves to serve Him in Kṛṣṇa consciousness, it will be possible at the time of death to transfer ourselves to the spiritual world and enter into Kṛṣṇaloka, Kṛṣṇa's planet, and enjoy ourselves in the association of Kṛṣṇa, the reservoir of all pleasure.

Kṛṣṇa's planet is described in the *Brahma-saṁhitā* (5.29) in this way:

cintāmaṇi-prakara-sadmasu kalpa-vṛkṣa-
lakṣāvṛteṣu surabhīr abhipālayantam
lakṣmī-sahasra-śata-sambhrama-sevyamānaṁ
govindam ādi-puruṣaṁ tam ahaṁ bhajāmi

"I worship Govinda, the primeval Lord, the first progenitor, who is tending the *surabhi* cows that fulfill all desires, who is surrounded by millions of purpose (wish-fulfilling) trees and abodes built with spiritual gems, and who is always served with great reverence and affection by hundreds and thousands of goddesses of fortune." In this way Kṛṣṇaloka is described. There the houses are made of touchstone (*cintāmaṇi*). If a small particle of touchstone touches an iron rod, that rod will immediately turn to gold. Of course, in this material world we have no experience with such a thing as touchstone, but according to the *Brahma-saṁhitā* all the abodes in Kṛṣṇaloka are composed of touchstone. Similarly, the trees there are called desire trees (*kalpa-vṛkṣa*) because one can get whatever he desires from them. Here we can get only mangoes from a mango tree, but in Kṛṣṇaloka we can get whatever we desire from any tree because the trees are *kalpa-vṛkṣa*. This is just a partial description of Kṛṣṇaloka, Kṛṣṇa's eternal abode in the spiritual sky.

The conclusion, therefore, is that we should not try to elevate ourselves to any material planet, because the same miserable conditions of birth, old age, disease, and death exist in all of them. Scientists are very proud of scientific advancement, but they have not been able to check old age, disease, and death. They can manufacture something to accelerate death, but nothing that can stop death. That is not within their power.

Those who are intelligent are interested in putting an end to birth, old age, disease, and death and entering into a spiritual life full of eternality, bliss, and knowledge. The *bhakti-yogī* knows that such a life is possible through practice of Kṛṣṇa consciousness and remembrance of Kṛṣṇa at the time of death.

> *ananya-cetāḥ satataṁ yo māṁ smarati nityaśaḥ*
> *tasyāhaṁ sulabhaḥ pārtha nitya-yuktasya yoginaḥ*

"For one who remembers Me without deviation, I am easy to obtain, O son of Pṛthā, because of his constant engagement in devotional service." (Bg. 8.14) In this verse the word *nitya-yukta* means "continuously in trance." Such a person who is continuously thinking of Kṛṣṇa and always engaged in Kṛṣṇa consciousness is the highest *yogī*. His attention is not diverted to *jñāna-yoga, dhyāna-yoga,* or any other system. For him, there is only one system—Kṛṣṇa consciousness. *Ananya-cetāḥ* means "without deviation." A Kṛṣṇa conscious devotee is not disturbed by anything, because his mind is always concentrated on Kṛṣṇa. The word *satatam* means that he is thinking of Kṛṣṇa at all places and at all times. When Kṛṣṇa descended onto this earth, He appeared in Vṛndāvana. Although I am presently living in America, my residence is in Vṛndāvana because I am always thinking of Kṛṣṇa. Although I may be in a New York apartment, my consciousness is there, and this is as good as being there.

Kṛṣṇa consciousness means always living with Kṛṣṇa on His spiritual planet. Because we are conscious of Kṛṣṇa, we are already living with Him. We simply have to wait to give up this material body to go there. For one who remembers Kṛṣṇa without deviation, He is easy to obtain. *Tasyāhaṁ sulabhaḥ pārtha:* "I become very cheap for them." For one who takes to Kṛṣṇa consciousness, the most valuable thing becomes very easy to obtain. Because one is engaged in *bhakti-yoga*, Kṛṣṇa becomes easily available. Why should we try so hard to attain Kṛṣṇa, when Kṛṣṇa Himself says, "I am easy to obtain"? We have only to chant Hare Kṛṣṇa, Hare Kṛṣṇa, Kṛṣṇa Kṛṣṇa, Hare Hare/ Hare Rāma, Hare Rāma, Rāma Rāma, Hare Hare twenty-four hours daily. There are no hard and fast rules and regulations. We can chant in the street or on the subway, in our home or in our office. There is neither expenditure nor tax.

Actually Kṛṣṇa, being omnipotent, is unconquerable, but it is said that He is not only obtained but conquered through pure devotional service. As stated before, it is generally very difficult to realize the Supreme Personality of Godhead; therefore one of His names is Ajita, meaning, "He whom no one can conquer." In *Śrīmad-Bhāgavatam* (10.14.3), Lord Brahmā prays to Ajita,

jñāne prayāsam udapāsya namanta eva
jīvanti san-mukharitāṁ bhavadīya-vārtām
sthāne sthitāḥ śruti-gatāṁ tanu-vāṅ-manobhir
ye prāyaśo 'jita jito 'py asi tais tri-lokyām

"O my dear Lord Ajita, those devotees who have thrown away the impersonal conceptions of the Absolute Truth and have therefore abandoned discussing empiric philosophical truths should hear from self-realized devotees about Your holy name, form, pastimes, and qualities. They should completely follow the principles of devotional service and remain free from illicit sex, gambling, intoxication, and animal slaughter. Surrendering themselves fully with body, words, and mind, they can live in any *āśrama* or social status. Indeed, You are conquered by such persons, although You are always unconquerable."

In this verse the words *jñāne prayāsam* refer to theosophists and philosophers who are trying year after year and life after life to understand God, or the Absolute Truth. Their attempts are like those of the frog in a well trying to comprehend the vastness of the Atlantic and Pacific oceans. Even our attempts to measure outer space are futile, to say nothing of the attempt to measure God. Such attempts are doomed to failure; therefore *Śrīmad-Bhāgavatam* recommends that we abandon all attempts to measure the Supreme. It is completely useless to try to understand God by our limited knowledge, and an intelligent man understands this. We should become submissive and try to understand that our position is very insignificant in this creation. The words *namanta eva* indicate that we are just to become submissive in order to understand the Supreme from a reliable source. And what is that source? *San-mukharitām:* from the lips of realized souls. Arjuna is understanding God directly from the lips of Kṛṣṇa, and we have to understand God through the lips of Arjuna or his bona fide representative. We can understand the transcendental nature of God only from a reliable source. That source may be Indian, European, American, Japanese, Hindu, Muslim, or whatever. The circumstances are not important. We just have to try to understand by hearing and then try to put the process into practice in our daily lives. By becoming submissive, hearing from the right source, and trying to apply the teachings in our daily lives, we can become conquerors of the Supreme. For one who does this, Lord Kṛṣṇa becomes easily available. Ordinarily, God realization is very difficult, but it is very easy for one who submissively hears (*śruti-gatām*).

There are two processes by which we can acquire knowledge: one is the ascending process (*āroha-panthā*), and the other is the descending process (*avaroha-panthā*). One who follows the ascending process attempts to understand God by his own efforts—by philosophizing, meditating, or speculating. One who follows the descending process acquires knowledge of God simply by hearing from an authority—from the bona fide spiritual master and the scriptures. As far as the ascending process is concerned, the *Brahma-saṁhitā* (5.34) states,

panthās tu koṭi-śata-vatsara-sampragamyo
vāyor athāpi manaso muni-puṅgavānām
so 'py asti yat-prapada-sīmny avicintya-tattve
govindam ādi-puruṣaṁ tam ahaṁ bhajāmi

"I worship Govinda, the primeval Lord, only the tips of the toes of whose lotus feet are approached by the *yogīs* and *jñānīs*, who travel for billions of years at the speed of the wind or mind." We can all understand how great the speed of the mind is. Although sitting in New York City, I can immediately think of India, which is thousands and thousands of miles away. It is herein stated that even if one travels at this speed for billions of years, Kṛṣṇa will still remain inconceivable. The word *muni-puṅgavānām* refers to a great thinker, not an ordinary man. Even if such a great thinker travels for millions of years at the speed of the mind, he will still find the Supreme Person unknowable. Yet for one who takes undeviatingly to this path of Kṛṣṇa consciousness, Kṛṣṇa is easy to obtain. Why is this? *Nitya-yuktasya yoginaḥ:* "Because such a person is constantly engaged in My devotional service, and I cannot forget him." So this is the process. We have only to become submissive to attract the attention of God. My Guru Mahārāja used to say, "Don't try to see God, but work in such a way that God will want to see you. God will take care of you. You don't have to *try* to see Him."

This should be our attitude. We should not think, "I want to see God. O God, please come and stand before me. Be my servant." But since God is no one's servant, we have to oblige Him by our love and service. We all know how difficult it is to see the king or president of a country. It is practically impossible for an ordinary man to get an interview with such an important person, to say nothing of having this important person come and stand before him. Yet people are demanding that the Supreme Personality of Godhead come and stand before them. It is our nature to hanker after Kṛṣṇa because He is the most attractive person in the universe—the most beautiful, most opulent, most powerful, most learned, most famous and most renounced. Everyone hankers after these qualities, and Kṛṣṇa is the reservoir of all of them—He possesses them in full. Kṛṣṇa is the reservoir of everything (*raso vai saḥ*); therefore when we hanker after beauty or power or knowledge or fame, we should just turn our attention to Kṛṣṇa. Then we will automatically get whatever our hearts desire.

10
The Path of Perfection

mām upetya punar janma duḥkhālayam aśāśvatam
nāpnuvanti mahātmānaḥ saṁsiddhiṁ paramāṁ gatāḥ

"After attaining Me, the great souls, who are *yogīs* in devotion, never return to this temporary world, which is full of miseries, because they have attained the highest perfection." (Bg. 8.15)

This material world is certified by its very creator, the Supreme Lord, as *duḥkhālayam*, which means "the place of miseries." Since this is the case, how can we possibly make it comfortable by so-called scientific advancement? *Duḥkha* means "misery" or "suffering," and real suffering is birth, old age, disease, and death. We have set these problems aside because we cannot solve them; therefore scientists concentrate on atomic bombs and spaceships. Why can't they solve these important problems that are always causing us to suffer? Obviously, they haven't the power to do so.

But in this verse, Śrī Kṛṣṇa gives the solution: *mām upetya punar janma . . . nāpnuvanti.* That is, "If one attains My platform, he does not come back again to this place of misery." Unfortunately, being in the mode of ignorance, people cannot understand that they are in a miserable situation. Animals cannot understand their miserable situations because they haven't the reasoning power. Man possesses reason whereby he can understand this, but in this age people are using their reasoning power to gratify their animal propensities. Reason should be used for getting liberated from this miserable condition. However, if we engage in Kṛṣṇa consciousness twenty-four hours a day without deviation, we will go to Kṛṣṇa and not be reborn in this miserable world. *Mahātmānaḥ saṁsiddhiṁ paramāṁ gatāḥ:* those great souls who have attained the highest perfection, Kṛṣṇa consciousness, are forever freed from misery. In this verse, the word *mahātmā* refers to a Kṛṣṇa conscious person eligible to enter the abode of Kṛṣṇa. The word *mahātmā* does not refer to a political leader like Mahatma Gandhi but to a great soul, a pure devotee of Kṛṣṇa.

When Kṛṣṇa says that the *mahātmā* enters His abode, He is referring to His transcendental kingdom, Goloka Vṛndāvana. The Vṛndāvana from which I have come is called Bhauma Vṛndāvana, which means it is the same Vṛndāvana descended on this earth. Just as Kṛṣṇa descended on this earth through His internal potency, similarly His *dhāma*, His abode, also descends. In other words, when Kṛṣṇa descends on this earth He manifests Himself in that particular land, Vṛndāvana, and therefore that land is also sacred. Apart from this, Kṛṣṇa has His own abode in the spiritual sky, and this is called Goloka Vṛndāvana.

The *mahātmā* prepares in this life to enter that transcendental abode. Human beings can utilize the facilities of nature to their best interest. Animals cannot. These facilities should be utilized in striving to become a *mahātmā* and putting an end to birth in this material world, which is characterized by the threefold miseries. The threefold miseries are those caused by the mind or body, by natural disturbances, and by other living entities. Whatever our position in this material world, there is always some kind of misery being inflicted upon us. Śrī Kṛṣṇa frankly says that it is not possible to avoid misery in this material world because this world is meant for misery. Unless miseries are present, we cannot come to Kṛṣṇa consciousness. Misery serves as an impetus to help elevate us to Kṛṣṇa consciousness. An intelligent person understands that although he does not want misery, miseries are being inflicted upon him by force. No one wants misery, but a person should be intelligent enough to ask, "Why are these miseries being forced upon me?" Unfortunately, people in the modern civilization try to set miseries aside, thinking, "Oh, why suffer? Let me cover my miseries with some intoxication." However, the miseries of life cannot be solved by artificial means such as intoxication. As soon as the intoxication is over, one returns to the same point. The miseries of material existence can be solved only by Kṛṣṇa consciousness. If we always remain in Kṛṣṇa consciousness, we'll be transferred to Kṛṣṇa's planet upon leaving this material body. That is the highest perfection.

People may inquire, "Well, you say that entering Kṛṣṇa's

planet constitutes the highest perfection, but we are interested in going to the moon. Is this not a kind of perfection?" Well, the desire to enter the higher planets is always there in the human mind. In fact, another name for the living entity is *sarva-gata,* which means that he wants to travel everywhere. That is the nature of the living entity. Americans who have money often go to India, Europe, or some other country because they do not like to stagnate in one place. That is our nature, and therefore we are interested in going to the moon or wherever. But according to Kṛṣṇa, even if we attain to the higher planets, we will still be subject to the material miseries.

ābrahma-bhuvanāl lokāḥ punar āvartino 'rjuna
mām upetya tu kaunteya punar janma na vidyate

"From the highest planet in the material world down to the lowest, all are places of misery wherein repeated birth and death take place. But one who attains to My abode, O son of Kuntī, never takes birth again." (Bg. 8.16)

The universe is divided into fourteen planetary systems (*caturdaśa-bhuvana*)—seven lower and seven higher. The earth is situated in the middle. In this verse Śrī Kṛṣṇa says, *ābrahma-bhuvanāl lokāḥ punar āvartinaḥ:* even if one enters the highest planet, Brahmaloka, there is still birth and death. The words *punar āvartinaḥ* mean "returning again," or "repetition of birth and death." We are changing bodies just as we change clothes, leaving one body and entering another. All planets are filled with living entities. We shouldn't think that only the earth is inhabited. There are living entities on the higher planets and lower planets as well. From our experience we can see that no place on earth is devoid of living entities. If we dig into the earth we find some worms, and if we go into the water we find many aquatics. The air is filled with birds, and if we analyze outer space we will find many living entities. It is illogical to conclude that there are no living entities on the other planets. To the contrary, they are *full* of living entities.

In any case, Kṛṣṇa says that from the highest planet to the lowest planet there is repetition of birth and death. Yet again, as in the former verse, He says, *mām upetya . . . punar janma na vidyate:* "If you reach My planet, you don't have to return to this miserable material world." To stress this point, Śrī Kṛṣṇa repeats it—that upon reaching Goloka Vṛndāvana, His eternal abode, one is liberated from the cycle of birth and death and attains eternal life. It is the duty of human life to understand these problems and attain a blissful, eternal life that is full of knowledge. Unfortunately, people in this age have forgotten the aim of life. Why? *Durāśayā ye bahir-artha-māninaḥ* (*Bhāg.* 7.5.31). People have been trapped by the material glitter—by skyscrapers, big factories, and political activities. People do not stop to consider that however big the skyscraper may be, they will not be allowed to live there indefinitely. We should not spoil our energy, therefore, in building great cities but should employ our energy for elevating ourselves to Kṛṣṇa consciousness. Kṛṣṇa consciousness is not a religious formula or some spiritual recreation but is the most important factor in our lives.

People are interested in attaining higher planets because there one's enjoyment is a thousand times greater and the duration of life much longer. As Kṛṣṇa says in the *Bhagavad-gītā* (8.17),

sahasra-yuga-paryantam ahar yad brahmaṇo viduḥ
rātriṁ yuga-sahasrāntāṁ te 'ho-rātra-vido janāḥ

"By human calculation, a thousand ages taken together form the duration of Brahmā's one day. And such also is the duration of his night."

The duration of the material universe is limited. It is manifested in cycles of *kalpas.* A *kalpa* is a day of Brahmā, and one day of Brahmā consists of a thousand cycles of four *yugas,* or ages: Satya, Tretā, Dvāpara, and Kali. The Age of Satya is characterized by virtue, wisdom, and religion, there being practically no ignorance and vice, and the *yuga* lasts 1,728,000 years. In the Tretā-yuga vice is introduced, and this *yuga* lasts 1,296,000 years. In the Dvāpara-yuga there is an even greater decline in virtue and religion, vice increasing, and this *yuga* lasts 864,000 years. And finally, in Kali-yuga (the *yuga* we have now been experiencing over the past 5,000 years), there is an abundance of strife, ignorance, irreligion, and vice, true virtue being practically nonexistent, and this *yuga* lasts 432,000 years. In Kali-yuga vice increases to such a point that at the termination of the *yuga* the Supreme Lord Himself appears as the Kalki-avatāra, vanquishes the demons, saves His devotees, and commences another Satya-yuga. Then the process is set rolling again. These four *yugas* rotating a thousand times constitute one day of Brahmā, the creator god, and the same number constitute one of his nights. Brahmā lives one hundred years comprised of such days and nights and then dies. By our calculations these hundred years total 311 trillion 40 billion earth years. Thus the life of Brahmā seems fantastic and interminable, but from the viewpoint of eternity it is as brief as a lightning flash. In the Causal Ocean there are innumerable Brahmās rising and disappearing like bubbles in the Atlantic. Brahmā and his creation are all part of the material universe, and therefore they are in constant flux.

In the material universe, not even Brahmā is free from the process of birth, old age, disease, and death. Brahmā, however, is directly engaged in the service of the Supreme Lord in the management of this universe; therefore he at once attains liberation at death. Elevated *sannyāsīs* are promoted to Brahmā's particular planet, Brahmaloka, which is the highest planet in the material universe and which, at the time of the partial annihilation, survives all the heavenly planets in the upper strata of the planetary system. Still, in due course Brahmā and all the other inhabitants of Brahmaloka are subject to death, according to the law of material nature. So even if we live millions and trillions of years, we have to die. Death cannot be avoided. Throughout the entire universe the process of creation and annihilation is taking place, as described in the next verse:

avyaktād vyaktayaḥ sarvāḥ prabhavanty ahar-āgame
rātry-āgame pralīyante tatraivāvyakta-saṁjñake

"At the beginning of Brahmā's day, all living entities become manifest from the unmanifest state, and thereafter, when the night falls, they are merged into the unmanifest again." (Bg. 8.18)

Unless we go to the spiritual sky, there is no escaping this process of birth and death, creation and annihilation. When Brahmā's days are finished, all the planets below Brahmaloka are covered by water, and when Brahmā rises again, creation takes place. The word *ahar* means "in the daytime," which is twelve hours of Brahmā's life. During this time this material manifestation—all these planets—are seen, but when night comes they are all merged in water. That is, they are annihilated. The word *rātry-āgame* means "at the fall of night." During this time, all these planets are invisible because they are inundated with water. This flux is the nature of the material world.

bhūta-grāmaḥ sa evāyaṁ bhūtvā bhūtvā pralīyate
rātry-āgame 'vaśaḥ pārtha prabhavaty ahar-āgame

"Again and again, when Brahmā's day arrives, all living entities come into being, and with the arrival of Brahmā's night they are helplessly annihilated." (Bg. 8.19) Although we do not want devastation, devastation is inevitable. At night, everything is flooded, and when day appears, gradually the waters disappear. For instance, on this one planet, the surface is three-fourths covered with water. Gradually, land is emerging, and the day will come when there will no longer be water but simply land. That is nature's process.

paras tasmāt tu bhāvo 'nyo 'vyakto 'vyaktāt sanātanaḥ
yaḥ sa sarveṣu bhūteṣu naśyatsu na vinaśyati

"Yet there is another unmanifest nature, which is eternal and is transcendental to this manifested and unmanifested matter. It is supreme and is never annihilated. When all in this world is annihilated, that part remains as it is." (Bg. 8.20)

We cannot calculate the length and breadth of this universe. There are millions and millions of universes like this within this material world, and above this material world is the spiritual sky, where the planets are all eternal. Life on those planets is also eternal. This material manifestation constitutes only one fourth of the entire creation. *Ekāṁśena sthito jagat. Ekāṁśena* means "one fourth." Three fourths of the creation is beyond this material sky, which is covered like a ball. This covering extends millions and millions of miles, and only after penetrating that covering can one enter the spiritual sky. That is open sky, eternal sky. In this verse it is stated, *paras tasmāt tu bhāvo 'nyaḥ:* "Yet there is another nature." The words *bhāvo 'nyaḥ* mean "another nature." We have experience only with this material nature, but from the *Bhagavad-gītā* we understand that there is a spiritual nature that is transcendental and eternal. We actually belong to that spiritual nature because we are spirit, but presently we are covered by this material body, and therefore we are a combination of matter and spirit. Just as we can understand that we are a combination of both natures, we should understand also that there is a spiritual world beyond this material universe. The spiritual nature is superior, and the material nature is inferior because matter cannot move without spirit.

This cannot be understood by experimental knowledge. We may look at millions and millions of stars through telescopes, but we cannot approach what we are seeing. Similarly, our senses are so insufficient that we cannot approach an understanding of the spiritual nature. Being incapable, we should not try to understand God and His kingdom by experimental knowledge. Rather, we have to understand by hearing the *Bhagavad-gītā.* There is no other way. If we want to know who our father is, we simply have to believe our mother. We have no way of knowing except from her. Similarly, in order to understand who God is and what His nature is, we have to accept the information given in the *Bhagavad-gītā.* There is no question of experimenting. Once we become advanced in Kṛṣṇa consciousness, we will realize God and His nature. We can come to understand, "Yes, there is God and a spiritual kingdom, and I have to go there. Indeed, I must prepare myself to go there."

The word *vyakta* means "manifest." This material universe that we are seeing (or partially seeing) before us is manifest. At least at night we can see that stars are twinkling and that there are innumerable planets. But beyond this *vyakta* is another nature, called *avyakta,* which is unmanifest. That is the spiritual nature, which is *sanātana,* eternal. This material nature has a beginning and an end, but that spiritual nature has neither beginning nor end. This material sky is within the covering of the *mahat-tattva,* matter. This matter is like a cloud. When there is a storm, it appears that the entire sky is covered with clouds, but actually only an insignificant part of the sky is covered. Because we are very minute, if just a few hundred miles are covered, it appears that the entire sky is covered. As soon as a wind comes and blows the clouds away, we can see the sky once again. Like the clouds, this *mahat-tattva* covering has a beginning and an end. Similarly, the material body, being a part of the material nature, has a beginning and an end. The body is born, grows, stays for some time, leaves some by-products, dwindles, and then vanishes. Whatever material manifestation we see undergoes these six basic transformations. Therefore whatever exists within material nature will ultimately be vanquished. But herein Kṛṣṇa is telling us that beyond this vanishing, cloudlike material nature is a superior nature, which is *sanātana*, eternal. *Yaḥ sa sarveṣu bhūteṣu naśyatsu na vinaśyati.* When this material manifestation is annihilated, that spiritual sky remains.

In the Second Canto of *Śrīmad-Bhāgavatam* we find a description of the spiritual sky and the people who live there. Its nature and features are also discussed. From the Second Canto we understand that there are spiritual airplanes in the spiritual sky and that the living entities there—who are all liberated—travel like lightning on those planes throughout the spiritual sky. This material world is simply an imitation; whatever we see here is simply a shadow of what exists there—something like what we see at the cinema, wherein we see but an imitation or a shadow of the real thing that is existing. As stated in *Śrīmad-Bhāgavatam* (1.1.1), *yatra tri-sargo 'mṛṣā:* "This material world is illusory." In store windows we often see mannequins, but no sane man thinks that these mannequins are real. He can see that they are imitations. Similarly, whatever we see here may be beautiful, just as a mannequin may be beautiful, but it is simply an imitation of the real beauty found in the spiritual world. As Śrīdhara Svāmī says, *yat satyatayā mithyā sargo 'pi satyavat pratīyate:* the spiritual world is real, and this unreal material manifestation only appears to be real. We must understand that reality will never be vanquished and that in essence reality means eternality. Therefore material pleasure, which is temporary, is not actual; real pleasure exists in Kṛṣṇa. Consequently, those who are after the reality don't participate in this shadow pleasure.

Thus when everything in the material world is annihilated, that spiritual nature remains eternally, and it is the purpose of human life to reach that spiritual sky. Unfortunately, people are not aware of the reality of the spiritual sky. According to *Śrīmad-Bhāgavatam* (7.5.31), *na te viduḥ svārtha-gatiṁ hi viṣṇum:* people do not know that their real self-interest lies in Viṣṇu, or Kṛṣṇa. They do not know that human life is meant for understanding spiritual reality and preparing oneself to be transferred to that reality. No one can remain here in this material world. All Vedic literatures instruct us in this way. *Tamasi mā jyotir gama:* "Don't remain in this darkness. Go to the light." According to Kṛṣṇa in the Fifteenth Chapter of the *Bhagavad-gītā* (15.6),

na tad bhāsayate sūryo na śaśāṅko na pāvakaḥ
yad gatvā na nivartante tad dhāma paramaṁ mama

"My abode is not illumined by the sun or moon, nor by electricity. One who reaches it never returns to this material world." This material world is dark by nature, and we are artificially illuminating it with electric lights, fire, and so on. In any case, its nature is dark, but the spiritual nature is full of light. When the sun is present, there is no darkness; similarly, every planet in the spiritual sky is self-luminous. Therefore there is no darkness, nor is there need of sun, moon, or electricity. The word *sūryo* means "sun," *śaśāṅko* means "moon," and *pāvakaḥ* means "fire" or "electricity." So these are not required in the spiritual sky for illumination. And again, Kṛṣṇa herein says, *yad gatvā na nivartante tad dhāma paramaṁ mama:* "That is My supreme abode, and one who reaches it never returns to this material world." This is stated throughout the *Bhagavad-gītā.* Again, in the Eighth Chapter (Bg. 8.21),

avyakto 'kṣara ity uktas tam āhuḥ paramāṁ gatim
yaṁ prāpya na nivartante tad dhāma paramaṁ mama

"That which the Vedāntists describe as unmanifest and infallible, that which is known as the supreme destination, that place from which, having attained it, one never returns—that is My supreme abode." Again, the word *avyakta,* meaning "unmanifest," is used. The word *akṣara* means "that which is never annihilated," or "that which is infallible." This means that since the supreme abode is eternal, it is not subject to the six transformations mentioned previously.

Because we are presently covered by a dress of material senses, we cannot see the spiritual world, and the spiritual nature is inconceivable for us. Yet we can *feel* that there is something spiritual present. Even a man completely ignorant of the spiritual nature can somehow feel its presence. One need only analyze his body silently: "What am I? Am I this finger? Am I this body? Am I this hair? No, I am not this, and I am not that. I am something other than this body. I am something beyond this body. What is that? That is the spiritual." In this way, we can feel or sense the presence of spirituality within this matter. We can sense the absence of spirit when a body is dead. If we witness someone dying, we can sense that something is leaving the body. Although we do not have the eyes to see it, that something is spirit. Its presence in the body is explained in the very beginning of the *Bhagavad-gītā* (2.17):

avināśi tu tad viddhi yena sarvam idaṁ tatam
vināśam avyayasyāsya na kaścit kartum arhati

"That which pervades the entire body you should know to be indestructible. No one is able to destroy that imperishable soul."

Spiritual existence is eternal, whereas the body is not. It is said that the spiritual atmosphere is *avyakta*, unmanifest. How, then, can it be manifest for us? Making the unmanifest manifest is the very process of Kṛṣṇa consciousness. According to the *Padma Purāṇa*,

ataḥ śrī-kṛṣṇa-nāmādi na bhaved grāhyam indriyaiḥ
sevonmukhe hi jihvādau svayam eva sphuraty adaḥ

"No one can understand Kṛṣṇa as He is by the blunt material senses. But He reveals Himself to the devotees, being pleased with them for their transcendental loving service unto Him." In this verse the word *indriyaiḥ* means "the senses." We have five senses for gathering knowledge (eyes, ears, nose, tongue, and skin), and five senses for working (voice, hands, legs, genitals, and anus). These ten senses are under the control of the mind. It is stated in this verse that with these dull material senses we cannot understand Kṛṣṇa's name, form, and so forth. Why is this? Because Kṛṣṇa is completely spiritual, and He is also absolute. Therefore His name, form, qualities, and paraphernalia are also spiritual. Due to material conditioning, or material bondage, we cannot presently understand what is spiritual, but this ignorance can be removed by chanting Hare Kṛṣṇa. If a man is sleeping, he can be awakened by sound vibration. You can call him, "Come on, it's time to get up!" Although the person is unconscious, hearing is so prominent that even a sleeping man can be awakened by sound vibration. Similarly, overpowered by this material conditioning, we are presently asleep to our spiritual consciousness, but we can be awakened to it by this transcendental vibration of Hare Kṛṣṇa, Hare Kṛṣṇa, Kṛṣṇa Kṛṣṇa, Hare Hare/ Hare Rāma, Hare Rāma, Rāma Rāma, Hare Hare. As stated before, *Hare* refers to the energy of the Lord, and *Kṛṣṇa* and *Rāma* refer to the Lord Himself. Therefore, when we chant Hare Kṛṣṇa, we are praying, "O Lord, O energy of the Lord, please accept me." We have no other prayer than "Please accept me." Lord Caitanya Mahāprabhu taught us that we should simply cry and pray that the Lord accept us. As Caitanya Mahāprabhu Himself prayed,

ayi nanda-tanuja kiṅkaraṁ
patitaṁ māṁ viṣame bhavāmbudhau
kṛpayā tava pāda-paṅkaja-
sthita-dhūlī-sadṛśaṁ vicintaya

"O Kṛṣṇa, son of Nanda, I am Your eternal servant, yet somehow or other I have fallen into this ocean of nescience and ignorance. Please pick Me up and place Me as one of the atoms at Your lotus feet." If a man has fallen into the ocean, his only hope for survival is that someone comes to pick him up. He only has to be lifted one inch above the water in order to feel immediate relief. Similarly, as soon as we take to Kṛṣṇa consciousness, we are lifted up, and we feel immediate relief.

We cannot doubt that the transcendental is there. The *Bhagavad-gītā* is being spoken by the Supreme Personality of Godhead Himself; therefore we should not doubt His words. The only problem is feeling and understanding what He is telling us. That understanding must be developed gradually, and that knowledge will be revealed by the chanting of Hare Kṛṣṇa. By this simple process we can come to understand the spiritual kingdom, the self, the material world, God, the nature of our conditioning, liberation from material bondage, and everything else. This is called *ceto-darpaṇa-mārjanam,* cleaning the dusty mirror of the impure mind.

Whatever the case, we must have faith in the words of Kṛṣṇa. When we purchase a ticket on Pan American or Air India, we have faith that that company will take us to our destination. Faith is created because the company is authorized. Our faith should not be blind; therefore we should accept that which is recognized. The *Bhagavad-gītā* has been recognized as authorized scripture in India for thousands of years, and even outside India there are many scholars, religionists, and philosophers who have accepted the *Bhagavad-gītā* as authoritative. It is said that even such a great scientist as Albert Einstein read the *Bhagavad-gītā* regularly. So we should not doubt the *Bhagavad-gītā's* authenticity.

Therefore when Lord Kṛṣṇa says that there is a supreme abode and that we can go there, we should have faith that such an abode exists. Many philosophers think that the spiritual abode is impersonal or void. Impersonalists like the Śaṅkarites and Buddhists generally speak of the void or emptiness, but the *Bhagavad-gītā* does not disappoint us in this way. The philosophy of voidism has simply created atheism, because it is the nature of the living entity to want enjoyment. As soon as he thinks that his future is void, he will try to enjoy the variegatedness of this material life. Thus impersonalism leads to armchair philosophical discussions and attachment to material enjoyment. We may enjoy speculating, but no real spiritual benefit can be derived from such speculation.

Bhaktiḥ pareśānubhavo viraktir anyatra ca (*Śrīmad-Bhāgavatam* 11.2.42). Once we have developed the devotional spirit, we will immediately become detached from all kinds of material enjoyment. As soon as a hungry man eats, he feels immediate satisfaction and says, "No, I don't want any more. I am satisfied." This satisfaction is a characteristic of the Kṛṣṇa conscious man.

brahma-bhūtaḥ prasannātmā na śocati na kāṅkṣati
samaḥ sarveṣu bhūteṣu mad-bhaktiṁ labhate parām

"One who is thus transcendentally situated at once realizes the Supreme Brahman and becomes fully joyful. He never laments or desires to have anything. He is equally disposed toward every living entity. In that state he attains pure devotional service unto Me." (Bg. 18.54)

As soon as one is spiritually realized, he feels full satisfaction and no longer hankers after flickering material enjoyment. As stated in the Second Chapter of the *Bhagavad-gītā* (2.59),

viṣayā vinivartante nirāhārasya dehinaḥ
rasa-varjaṁ raso 'py asya paraṁ dṛṣṭvā nivartate

"Although the embodied soul may be restricted from sense enjoyment, the taste for sense objects remains. But ceasing such engagements by experiencing a higher taste, he is fixed in consciousness." A doctor may tell a diseased man, "Don't eat this. Don't eat that. Don't have sex. Don't. Don't." In this way a diseased man is forced to accept so many "don'ts," but inside he is thinking, "Oh, if I can just get these things, I'll be happy." The desires remain inside. However, when one is established in Kṛṣṇa consciousness, he is so strong inside that he doesn't experience the desire. Although he's not impotent, he doesn't want sex. He can marry thrice but still be detached. *Paraṁ dṛṣṭvā nivartate.* When something superior is acquired, one naturally gives up all inferior things. That which is superior is the Supreme Personality of Godhead, and atheism and impersonalism cannot give us this. He is attained only by unalloyed devotion.

puruṣaḥ sa paraḥ pārtha bhaktyā labhyas tv ananyayā
yasyāntaḥ-sthāni bhūtāni yena sarvam idaṁ tatam

"The Supreme Personality of Godhead, who is greater than all, is attainable by unalloyed devotion. Although He is present in His abode, He is all-pervading, and everything is situated within Him." (Bg. 8.22) The words *puruṣaḥ sa paraḥ* indicate the Supreme Person, Kṛṣṇa, who is greater than all others. This is not a void speaking, but a person who has all the characteristics of personality in full. Just as we are talking face to face, when we reach the supreme abode we can talk to God face to face. We can play with Him, eat with Him, and do everything else. This state is not acquired by mental speculation but by transcendental loving service (*bhaktyā labhyaḥ*). The words *tv ananyayā* indicate that this *bhakti* must be without adulteration. It must be unalloyed.

Although the Supreme Personality is a person and is present in His abode in the spiritual sky, He is so widespread that everything is within Him. He is both inside and outside. Although God is everywhere, He still has His kingdom, His abode. The sun may pervade the universe with its sunshine, yet the sun itself is a separate entity.

In His supreme abode, the Supreme Lord has no rival. Wherever we may be, we find a predominating personality. In the United States, the predominating personality is the President. However, when the next election comes, the President will have so many rivals, but in the spiritual sky the Supreme Lord has no rival. Those who want to become His rivals are placed in this material world, under the conditions of material nature. In the spiritual sky there is no rivalry, and all the inhabitants there are liberated souls. From *Śrīmad-Bhāgavatam* we receive information that their bodily features resemble God's. In some of the spiritual planets God manifests a two-armed form, and in others He manifests a four-armed form. The living entities of those planets have corresponding features, and one cannot distinguish who is God and who is not. This is called *sārūpya-mukti* liberation, wherein one has the same features as the Lord. There are five kinds of liberation: *sāyujya, sārūpya, sālokya, sārṣṭi,* and *sāmīpya. Sāyujya-mukti* means merging into God's impersonal effulgence, the *brahmajyoti.* As we have discussed, the attempt to merge into the *brahmajyoti* and lose individuality is not desirable and is very risky. *Sārūpya-mukti* means attaining a body exactly like God's. *Sālokya-mukti* means living on the same planet with God. *Sārṣṭi-mukti* means having the opulence of God. For instance, God is very powerful, and we can become powerful like Him. That is called *sārṣṭi. Sāmīpya-mukti* means always remaining with God as one of His associates. For instance, Arjuna is always with Kṛṣṇa as His friend, and this is called *sāmīpya-mukti.* We can attain any one of these five types of liberation, but out of these five, *sāyujya-mukti,* merging into the *brahmajyoti,* is rejected by Vaiṣṇava philosophy. According to the Vaiṣṇava philosophy, we worship God as He is and retain our separate identity eternally in order to serve Him. According to the Māyāvāda philosophy, impersonalism, one tries to lose his individual identity and merge into the existence of the Supreme. That, however, is a suicidal policy and is not recommended by Kṛṣṇa in the *Bhagavad-gītā.*

This has also been rejected by Lord Caitanya Mahāprabhu, who advocated worship in separation. As stated before, the pure devotee does not even want liberation; he simply asks to remain Kṛṣṇa's devotee birth after birth. This is Lord Caitanya Mahāprabhu's prayer, and the words "birth after birth" indicate that the pure devotee doesn't care whether he is liberated or not. He simply wants to engage in Kṛṣṇa consciousness, to serve the Supreme Lord. Always wanting to engage in God's transcendental loving service is the symptom of pure devotion. Of course, wherever a devotee is, he remains in the spiritual kingdom, even though in the material body. On his part, he does not demand any of the five types of liberation, nor anything for his personal superiority or comfort. But in order to associate with God in the spiritual planets, one must become His pure devotee.

For those who are not pure devotees, Lord Kṛṣṇa explains at what times one should leave the body in order to attain liberation.

> *yatra kāle tv anāvṛttim āvṛttiṁ caiva yoginaḥ*
> *prayātā yānti taṁ kālaṁ vakṣyāmi bharatarṣabha*

"O best of the Bhāratas, I shall now explain to you the different times at which, passing away from this world, the *yogī* does or does not come back." (Bg. 8.23) In India, unlike in the West, it is common for astrologers to make minute calculations of the astronomical situation at the moment of one's birth. Indeed, a person's horoscope is read not only when he is born but also when he dies, in order to determine what his situation will be in the next life. All this can be determined by astrological calculation. In this verse, Lord Kṛṣṇa is accepting those astrological principles, confirming that if one leaves his body at a particular time he may attain liberation. If one dies at one moment he may be liberated, and if he dies at another moment he may have to return to the material world. It is all a question of chance. For the devotee, however, there is no question of chance. Whatever the astrological situation, the devotee in

Kṛṣṇa consciousness is guaranteed liberation. For others there are chances that if they leave their body at a particular moment they may attain liberation and enter the spiritual kingdom, or they may be reborn.

agnir jyotir ahaḥ śuklaḥ ṣaṇ-māsā uttarāyaṇam
tatra prayātā gacchanti brahma brahma-vido janāḥ

"Those who know the Supreme Brahman attain that Supreme by passing away from the world during the influence of the fiery god, in the light, at an auspicious moment of the day, during the fortnight of the waxing moon, or during the six months when the sun travels in the north." (Bg. 8.24) As we all know, six months out of the year the sun shines most directly north of the equator, and six months south. So if a person dies when the sun is in the northern hemisphere, he can attain liberation. That is not only the verdict of the *Bhagavad-gītā,* but also of other scriptures.

dhūmo rātris tathā kṛṣṇaḥ ṣaṇ-māsā dakṣiṇāyanam
tatra cāndramasaṁ jyotir yogī prāpya nivartate

"The mystic who passes away from this world during the smoke, the night, the fortnight of the waning moon, or the six months when the sun passes to the south reaches the moon planet but again comes back." (Bg. 8.25) No one can say when he is going to die, and in that sense the moment of one's death is accidental. However, for a devotee in Kṛṣṇa consciousness, there is no question of accident.

śukla-kṛṣṇe gatī hy ete jagataḥ śāśvate mate
ekayā yāty anāvṛttim anyayāvartate punaḥ

"According to the *Vedas,* there are two ways of passing from this world—one in light and one in darkness. When one passes in light, he does not come back, but when one passes in darkness, he returns." (Bg. 8.26) The same description of departure and return is quoted by Ācārya Baladeva Vidyābhūṣaṇa from the *Chāndogya Upaniṣad.* In such a way, those who are fruitive laborers and philosophical speculators from time immemorial are constantly going and coming. Actually they do not attain ultimate salvation, for they do not surrender to Kṛṣṇa.

naite sṛtī pārtha jānan yogī muhyati kaścana
tasmāt sarveṣu kāleṣu yoga-yukto bhavārjuna

"Although the devotees know these two paths, O Arjuna, they are never bewildered. Therefore be always fixed in devotion." (Bg. 8.27) Herein the Lord confirms that there is no question of chance for one who practices *bhakti-yoga*. His destination is certain. Whether he dies when the sun is in the northern or southern hemisphere is of no importance. As we have already stated, one who thinks of Kṛṣṇa at the time of death will at once be transferred to Kṛṣṇa's abode. Therefore Kṛṣṇa tells Arjuna to always remain in Kṛṣṇa consciousness. This is possible through the chanting of Hare Kṛṣṇa. Since Kṛṣṇa and His spiritual kingdom are nondifferent, being absolute, Kṛṣṇa and His sound vibration are the same. Simply by vibrating Kṛṣṇa's name, we can enjoy Kṛṣṇa's association. If we are walking down the street chanting Hare Kṛṣṇa, Kṛṣṇa is going with us. If we walk down the street and look up at the sky, we may see that the sun or the moon is accompanying us. I can recall about fifty years ago, when I was a householder, my second son, who was about four years old at the time, was walking with me down the street, and he suddenly asked me, "Father, why is the moon going with us?"

If a material object like the moon has the power to accompany us, we can surely understand that the Supreme Lord, who is all-powerful, can always remain with us. Being omnipotent, He can always keep us company, provided that we are qualified to keep His company. Pure devotees are always merged in the thought of Kṛṣṇa and are always remembering that Kṛṣṇa is with them. Lord Caitanya Mahāprabhu has confirmed the absolute nature of Kṛṣṇa in His *Śikṣāṣṭaka* (verse 2):

nāmnām akāri bahudhā nija-sarva-śaktis
tatrārpitā niyamitaḥ smaraṇe na kālaḥ
etādṛśī tava kṛpā bhagavan mamāpi
durdaivam īdṛśam ihājani nānurāgaḥ

"My Lord, O Supreme Personality of Godhead, in Your holy name there is all good fortune for the living entity, and therefore You have many names, such as Kṛṣṇa and Govinda, by which You expand Yourself. You have invested all Your potencies in those names, and there are no hard-and-fast rules for remembering them. My dear Lord, although You bestow such mercy upon the fallen, conditioned souls by liberally teaching Your holy names, I am so unfortunate that I commit offenses while chanting the holy name, and therefore I do not achieve attachment for chanting."

We may take the effort to spend a great deal of money and attempt to build or establish a temple for Kṛṣṇa, but if we do so we must observe many rules and regulations and see properly to the temple's management. But herein it is confirmed that simply by chanting Hare Kṛṣṇa, any man can have the benefit of keeping company with Kṛṣṇa. Just as Arjuna is deriving benefit by being in the same chariot with Lord Śrī Kṛṣṇa, we can also benefit by associating with Kṛṣṇa through the chanting of His holy names—Hare Kṛṣṇa, Hare Kṛṣṇa, Kṛṣṇa Kṛṣṇa, Hare Hare/ Hare Rāma, Hare Rāma, Rāma Rāma, Hare Hare. This *mahā-mantra* is not my personal concoction but is authorized by Lord Caitanya Mahāprabhu, who is not only an authority but the incarnation of Lord Śrī Kṛṣṇa Himself.

Although the *mahā-mantra* is in the Sanskrit language and many people do not know its meaning, it is still so attractive that people participate when it is chanted publicly. When chanting the *mahā-mantra*, we are completely safe, even in the most dangerous position. We should always be aware that in this material world we are always in a dangerous position. *Śrīmad-Bhāgavatam* confirms: *padaṁ padaṁ yad vipadām.* In this world, there is danger at every step. The devotees of the Lord, however, are not meant to remain in this miserable, dangerous place. Therefore we should take care to advance in Kṛṣṇa consciousness while in this human form. Then our happiness is assured.

PART TWO: THE PERFECTION OF YOGA

1
Yoga as Rejected by Arjuna

There have been many *yoga* systems popularized in the Western world, especially in this century, but none of them have actually taught the perfection of *yoga*. In the *Bhagavad-gītā* Śrī Kṛṣṇa, the Supreme Personality of Godhead, directly teaches Arjuna the perfection of *yoga*. If we actually want to participate in the perfection of the *yoga* system, in *Bhagavad-gītā* we will find the authoritative statements of the Supreme Person.

It is certainly remarkable that the perfection of *yoga* was taught in the middle of a battlefield. It was taught to Arjuna, a warrior, just before he was to engage in a fratricidal battle. Out of sentiment Arjuna was thinking, "Why should I fight against my own kinsmen?" That reluctance to fight was due to Arjuna's illusion, and just to eradicate that illusion Śrī Kṛṣṇa spoke the *Bhagavad-gītā* to him. One can just imagine how little time must have elapsed while the *Bhagavad-gītā* was being spoken. All the warriors on both sides were poised to fight, so there was very little time indeed—at the utmost, one hour. Within this one hour the whole the *Bhagavad-gītā* was discussed, and Śrī Kṛṣṇa set forth the perfection of all *yoga* systems to His friend Arjuna. At the end of this great discourse, Arjuna set aside his misgivings and fought.

However, within the discourse, when Arjuna heard the explanation of the meditational system of *yoga*—how to sit down, how to keep the body straight, how to keep the eyes half-closed, and how to gaze at the tip of the nose without diverting one's attention, all this being conducted in a secluded place, alone—he replied,

> *yo 'yaṁ yogas tvayā proktaḥ sāmyena madhusūdana*
> *etasyāhaṁ na paśyāmi cañcalatvāt sthitiṁ sthirām*

"O Madhusūdana, the system of *yoga* You have summarized

appears impractical and unendurable to me, for the mind is restless and unsteady." (Bg. 6.33) This is important. We must always remember that we are in a material circumstance wherein at every moment our mind is subject to agitation. Actually we are not in a very comfortable situation. We are always thinking that by changing our situation we will overcome our mental agitation, and we are always thinking that when we reach a certain point, all mental agitations will disappear. But it is the nature of the material world that we cannot be free from anxiety. Our dilemma is that although we are always trying to make a solution to our problems, this universe is so designed that these solutions never come.

Not being a cheater, being very frank and open, Arjuna tells Kṛṣṇa that the system of *yoga* He has described is not possible for him to execute. In speaking to Kṛṣṇa, it is significant that Arjuna addresses Him as Madhusūdana, indicating that the Lord is the killer of the demon Madhu. It is notable that God's names are innumerable, for He is often named according to His activities. Indeed, God has innumerable names because He has innumerable activities. We are only parts of God, and we cannot even remember how many activities we have engaged in from our childhood to the present. The eternal God is unlimited, and since His activities are also unlimited, He has unlimited names, of which *Kṛṣṇa* is the chief. Then why is Arjuna addressing Him as Madhusūdana when, being Kṛṣṇa's friend, he could address Him directly as Kṛṣṇa? The answer is that Arjuna considers his mind to be like a great demon, such as the demon Madhu. If it were possible for Kṛṣṇa to kill the demon called the mind, then Arjuna would be able to attain the perfection of *yoga*. "My mind is much stronger than this demon Madhu," Arjuna is saying. "Please, if You could kill him, then it would be possible for me to execute this *yoga* system." Even the mind of a great man like Arjuna is always agitated. As Arjuna himself says,

cañcalaṁ hi manaḥ kṛṣṇa pramāthi balavad dṛḍham
tasyāhaṁ nigrahaṁ manye vāyor iva suduṣkaram

"The mind is restless, turbulent, obstinate, and very strong, O Kṛṣṇa, and to subdue it, I think, is more difficult than controlling the wind." (Bg. 6.34)

It is indeed a fact that the mind is always telling us to go here, go there, do this, do that—it is always telling us which way to turn. Thus the sum and substance of the *yoga* system is to control the agitated mind. In the meditational *yoga* system the mind is controlled by focusing it on the Supersoul—that is the whole purpose of *yoga.* But Arjuna says that controlling the mind is more difficult than stopping the wind from blowing. One can imagine a man stretching out his arms to try to stop a hurricane. Are we to assume that Arjuna is simply not sufficiently qualified to control his mind? The actual fact is that we cannot begin to understand the immense qualifications of Arjuna. After all, he was a personal friend of the Supreme Personality of Godhead. This is a highly elevated position and is one that cannot be at all attained by one without great qualifications. In addition to this, Arjuna was renowned as a great warrior and administrator. He was such an intelligent man that he could understand the *Bhagavad-gītā* within one hour, whereas at the present moment great scholars cannot even understand it in the course of a lifetime. Yet Arjuna was thinking that controlling the mind was simply not possible for him. Are we then to assume that what was impossible for Arjuna in a more advanced age is possible for us in this degenerate age? We should not for one moment think that we are in Arjuna's category. We are a thousand times inferior.

Moreover, there is no record of Arjuna's having executed the *yoga* system at any time. Yet Arjuna was praised by Kṛṣṇa as the only man worthy of understanding the *Bhagavad-gītā.* What was Arjuna's great qualification? Śrī Kṛṣṇa says, "You are My devotee. You are My very dear friend." Despite this qualification, Arjuna refused to execute the meditational *yoga* system described by Śrī Kṛṣṇa. What then are we to conclude? Are we to despair the mind's ever being controlled? No, it can be controlled, and the process is Kṛṣṇa consciousness. The mind must always be fixed on Kṛṣṇa. Insofar as our mind is absorbed in thoughts of Kṛṣṇa, we have attained the perfection of *yoga.*

Now, when we turn to *Śrīmad-Bhāgavatam,* in the Twelfth Canto we find Śukadeva Gosvāmī telling Mahārāja Parīkṣit that in the golden age, the Satya-yuga, people lived for one hundred thousand years and thus it was possible for such advanced beings to execute this meditational system of *yoga.* But what was achieved in Satya-yuga by this meditational process, and in the following *yuga,* Tretā-yuga, by the offering of great sacrifices, and in the next *yuga,* Dvāpara-yuga, by temple worship, can be achieved at the present time, in Kali-yuga, by simply chanting the names of God, *hari-kīrtana,* Hare Kṛṣṇa. So from authoritative sources we learn that the chanting of Hare Kṛṣṇa, Hare Kṛṣṇa, Kṛṣṇa Kṛṣṇa, Hare Hare/ Hare Rāma, Hare Rāma, Rāma Rāma, Hare Hare is the embodiment of the perfection of *yoga* for this age.

Today we have great difficulty living fifty or sixty years. A man may live at the utmost eighty or a hundred years. In addition, these brief years are always fraught with anxiety, with difficulties due to circumstances of war, pestilence, and famine, and with so many other disturbances. We're also not very intelligent, and at the same time we're unfortunate. These are the characteristics of people living in Kali-yuga, the present degraded age. So properly speaking, we can never attain success in the meditational *yoga* system described by Kṛṣṇa.

At the utmost we can only gratify our personal whims by some pseudo adaptation of this system. Thus people are paying money to attend some classes in gymnastic exercises and deep breathing, and they're happy if they think they can lengthen their lifetimes by a few years or enjoy better sex life. But we must understand that this is not the actual *yoga* system. In this age that meditational system cannot be properly executed. Instead, all of the perfections of that system can be realized through *bhakti-yoga,* the sublime process of Kṛṣṇa consciousness, specifically *mantra-yoga,* the glorification of Śrī Kṛṣṇa through the chanting of Hare Kṛṣṇa. That is recommended in the Vedic scriptures and has been introduced by great authorities like Caitanya Mahāprabhu. Indeed, the *Bhagavad-gītā* proclaims that the *mahātmās,* the great souls, are always chanting the glories of the Lord. If one wants to be a *mahātmā* in terms of the Vedic literature, in terms of the *Bhagavad-gītā,* and in terms of the great authorities, then one has to adopt the process of Kṛṣṇa consciousness, beginning with the chanting of Hare Kṛṣṇa. But if we're content with making a show of meditation by sitting very straight in the lotus position and going into a trance like some sort of performer, then that is a different thing. We should understand, however, that such show-bottle performances have nothing to do with the actual perfection of *yoga.* The material disease cannot be cured by artificial medicine. We have to take the real cure straight from Kṛṣṇa.

2

Yoga as Work in Devotion

We have heard the names of so many different *yogas* and *yogīs*, but in the *Bhagavad-gītā* Kṛṣṇa says that the actual *yogī* is he who has surrendered himself "fully unto Me." Kṛṣṇa also proclaims that there is no difference between renunciation (*sannyāsa*) and *yoga:*

yaṁ sannyāsam iti prāhur yogaṁ taṁ viddhi pāṇḍava
na hy asannyasta-saṅkalpo yogī bhavati kaścana

"What is called renunciation you should know to be the same as *yoga,* or linking oneself with the Supreme, O son of Pāṇḍu, for one can never become a *yogī* unless he renounces the desire for sense gratification." (Bg. 6.2)

In the *Bhagavad-gītā* there are four basic types of *yoga* delineated—*karma-yoga, jñāna-yoga, dhyāna-yoga,* and *bhakti-yoga.* The systems of *yoga* may be likened to a staircase. Someone may be on the first step, someone may be halfway up, or someone may be on the top step. When one is elevated to certain levels, he is known as a *karma-yogī, jñāna-yogī,* etc. All these *yogas* aim at realization of the Supreme, and the culmination is *bhakti-yoga,* devotional service to the Supreme Lord..

Some *yogīs* perform *yoga* for a profit, but that is not real *yoga.* Everything must be engaged in the service of the Lord. Whatever we do as an ordinary worker or as a *sannyāsī* or as a *yogī* or as a philosopher must be done in Kṛṣṇa consciousness. When we are absorbed in the thought of serving Kṛṣṇa and when we act in that consciousness, we can become real *sannyāsīs* and real *yogīs.* For those who are taking the first step up the staircase of the *yoga* system, there is work. One should not think that simply because he is beginning *yoga* he should stop working. In the *Bhagavad-gītā* Kṛṣṇa asks Arjuna to become a *yogī,* but He never tells him to cease from fighting.

Quite the contrary. Of course, one may ask how a person may be a *yogī* and at the same time a warrior. Our conception of *yoga* practice is that of sitting very straight, with legs crossed and eyes half-closed, staring at the tip of our nose and concentrating in this way in a lonely place. So how is it that Kṛṣṇa is asking Arjuna to become a *yogī* and at the same time participate in a ghastly civil war? That is the mystery of the *Bhagavad-gītā:* one can remain a fighting man and at the same time be the highest *yogī*, the highest *sannyāsī.* How is this possible? In Kṛṣṇa consciousness. One simply has to fight for Kṛṣṇa, work for Kṛṣṇa, eat for Kṛṣṇa, sleep for Kṛṣṇa, and dedicate all activities to Kṛṣṇa. In this way one becomes the highest *yogī* and the highest *sannyāsī.* That is the secret.

In the Sixth Chapter of the *Bhagavad-gītā*, Śrī Kṛṣṇa instructs Arjuna how to perform meditational *yoga*, but Arjuna rejects this as too difficult. How then is Arjuna considered to be a great *yogī*? Although Kṛṣṇa saw that Arjuna was rejecting the meditational system, He proclaimed Arjuna to be the highest *yogī* because "You are always thinking of Me." Thinking of Kṛṣṇa is the essence of all *yoga* systems—of *karma-*, *jñāna-*, *dhyāna-*, or *bhakti-yoga* or any other system of *yoga*, sacrifice, or charity. All the recommended activities for spiritual realization end in Kṛṣṇa consciousness, in thinking always of Kṛṣṇa. The actual perfection of human life lies in being always Kṛṣṇa conscious and always being aware of Kṛṣṇa while performing all types of activities.

In the preliminary stage one is advised to always work for Kṛṣṇa. One must be always searching out some duty or some engagement, for it is a bad policy to remain idle even for a second. When one actually becomes advanced through such engagements, he may not work physically, but he is always engaged within by constantly thinking of Kṛṣṇa. In the preliminary stage, however, one is always advised to engage one's senses in the service of Kṛṣṇa. There are a variety of activities one can perform in serving Kṛṣṇa. The International Society for Krishna Consciousness is intended to help direct aspirant devotees in these activities. for those working in Kṛṣṇa consciousness, there are simply not enough hours in the day to serve Kṛṣṇa. There are always activities, engagements both day and night, which the student of Kṛṣṇa consciousness performs joyfully. That is the stage of real happiness—constant engagement for Kṛṣṇa and spreading Kṛṣṇa consciousness around the world. In the material world one may become very tired if he works all the time, but if one works in Kṛṣṇa consciousness, he can chant Hare Kṛṣṇa and engage in devotional service twenty-four hours a day and never get tired. But if we vibrate some mundane sound, we soon become exhausted. There is no question of becoming tired on the spiritual platform, because the spiritual platform is absolute. In the material world everyone is working for sense gratification, and therefore the profits of one's labor are used to gratify one's senses. But a real *yogī* does not desire such fruits. He has no desire other than Kṛṣṇa.

3
Yoga as Meditation on Kṛṣṇa

In India there are sacred places where *yogīs* go to meditate in solitude, as prescribed in the *Bhagavad-gītā*. Traditionally, *yoga* cannot be executed in a public place, but insofar as *kīrtana* is concerned—that is, *mantra-yoga*, or the *yoga* of chanting the Hare Kṛṣṇa *mantra:* Hare Kṛṣṇa, Hare Kṛṣṇa, Kṛṣṇa Kṛṣṇa, Hare Hare/ Hare Rāma, Hare Rāma, Rāma Rāma, Hare Hare—the more people present, the better. When Lord Caitanya Mahāprabhu was performing *kīrtana* in India some five hundred years ago, He organized sixteen people in each group to lead the chanting, and thousands of people chanted with them. This participation in *kīrtana,* in the public chanting of the names and glories of God, is very easy in this age, but the meditational process of *yoga* is very difficult. It is specifically stated in the *Bhagavad-gītā* that to perform meditational *yoga* one should go to a secluded and holy place. In other words, it is necessary to leave home. In this age it is not always possible to go to a secluded, holy place, but this is not necessary in *bhakti-yoga.*

In the *bhakti-yoga* system there are nine different processes: hearing, chanting, remembering, serving, worshiping the Deity in the temple, praying, carrying out Kṛṣṇa's orders, serving Kṛṣṇa as a friend, and sacrificing everything for Him. Out of these, *śravaṇaṁ kīrtanam,* hearing and chanting, are the most important. At a public *kīrtana* one person can chant Hare Kṛṣṇa, Hare Kṛṣṇa, Kṛṣṇa Kṛṣṇa, Hare Hare/ Hare Rāma, Hare Rāma, Rāma Rāma, Hare Hare while a group listens, and at the end of the *mantra* the group can respond, and in this way there is a reciprocation of hearing and chanting. This can easily be performed in one's own home with a small group of friends, or in a large public place with many people. On the other hand, while one may attempt to practice meditational *yoga* in a large city, one must understand that this is one's own concoction and is not the method recommended in the *Bhagavad-gītā.*

The whole purpose of *yoga* is to purify oneself. And what is this purification? Purification means realizing one's actual identity, that "I am pure spirit—I am not matter." Due to material contact, we are identifying ourselves with matter and thinking, "I am this body." But by performing real *yoga* one realizes his constitutional position as being distinct from matter. The purpose of seeking out a secluded place and executing the meditational process is to help one come to this understanding. It is not possible to come to this understanding if one executes the process improperly. In any case, Lord Caitanya Mahāprabhu has declared:

harer nāma harer nāma harer nāmaiva kevalam
kalau nāsty eva nāsty eva nāsty eva gatir anyathā

"In this age of quarrel and disagreement [Kali-yuga], the only way of spiritual realization is the chanting of the names of Kṛṣṇa. There is no other way, there is no other way, there is no other way."

It is generally thought, at least in the Western world, that the *yoga* system involves meditating on the void. But the Vedic literatures do not recommend meditating on any void. Rather, the *Vedas* maintain that *yoga* means meditation on Viṣṇu, and this is also maintained in the *Bhagavad-gītā.* In many *yoga* societies we find that people sit cross-legged and very straight, then close their eyes to meditate, and so fifty percent of them go to sleep, because when we close our eyes and have no subject matter for contemplation, we simply go to sleep. Of course, this is not recommended by Śrī Kṛṣṇa in the *Bhagavad-gītā.* One must sit very straight, with the eyes only half-closed, gazing at the tip of the nose. If one does not follow the instructions, the result will be sleep and nothing more. Sometimes, of course, meditation goes on when one is sleeping, but this is not the recommended process for the execution of *yoga.* Thus, Kṛṣṇa advises that to keep oneself awake one should always keep the tip of the nose visible. In addition, one must always remain undisturbed. If the mind is agitated or if there is a great deal of activity going on, one will not be able to concentrate. In meditational *yoga* one must also be devoid of fear. There must be no question of fear when one enters spiritual life. And one must also be completely free from sex life. Nor can there be any demands on one meditating in this way. When there are no demands and one executes this system properly, then he can control his mind. After one has met all the requirements for meditation, he must transfer his whole thought to Kṛṣṇa, or Viṣṇu. It is not that one is to transfer his thought to vacancy. Thus Kṛṣṇa says that one absorbed in the meditational *yoga* system is "always thinking of Me."

The *yogī* obviously has to go through a great deal of difficulty to purify the *ātmā* (mind, body, and soul), but it is a fact that this can be done most effectively in this age simply by the chanting of Hare Kṛṣṇa, Hare Kṛṣṇa, Kṛṣṇa Kṛṣṇa, Hare Hare/ Hare Rāma, Hare Rāma, Rāma Rāma, Hare Hare. Why is this? Because this transcendental sound vibration is nondifferent from Kṛṣṇa. When we chant His name with devotion, then Kṛṣṇa is with us, and when Kṛṣṇa is with us, then what is the possibility of remaining impure? Consequently, one absorbed in Kṛṣṇa consciousness, in chanting the names of Kṛṣṇa and serving Him always, receives the benefit of the highest form of *yoga.* The advantage is that he doesn't have to take all the trouble of the meditational process. That is the beauty of Kṛṣṇa consciousness.

In *yoga* it is necessary to control all of the senses, and when all the senses are controlled, the mind must be engaged in thinking of Viṣṇu. One becomes peaceful after thus conquering material life: *jitātmanaḥ praśāntasya paramātmā samāhitaḥ.* "For one who has conquered the mind, the Supersoul is already reached, for he has attained tranquillity." (Bg. 6.7) This material world has been likened to a great forest fire. As in the forest a fire may automatically take place, so in this material world, although we may try to live peacefully, there is always a great conflagration. It is not possible to live in peace anywhere in the material world. But for one who is transcendentally situated—either by the meditational *yoga* system or by the empirical philosophical method or by *bhakti-yoga*—peace is possible. All forms of *yoga* are meant for transcendental life, but the method of chanting is especially effective in this age. *Kīrtana* may go on for hours and one will not feel tired, but it is difficult to sit in the lotus position perfectly still for more than a few minutes. Yet regardless of the process, once the fire of material life is extinguished, one does not simply experience what is called the impersonal void. Rather, as Kṛṣṇa tells Arjuna, one enters into the supreme abode:

yuñjann evaṁ sadātmānaṁ yogī niyata-mānasaḥ
śāntiṁ nirvāṇa-paramāṁ mat-saṁsthām adhigacchati

"By meditating in this manner, always controlling the body, mind, and activities, the mystic transcendentalist attains to the kingdom of God through the cessation of material existence." (Bg. 6.15) Kṛṣṇa's abode is not void. It is like an establishment, and in an establishment there is a variety of engagements. The successful *yogī* actually attains to the kingdom of God, where there is spiritual variegatedness. The *yoga* processes are simply ways to elevate oneself to enter into that abode. Actually we belong to that abode, but being forgetful, we have been put into this material world. Just as a madman becomes crazy and is put into a lunatic asylum, so we, losing sight of our spiritual identity, become crazy and are put into this material world. Thus the material world is a sort of lunatic asylum, and we can easily notice that nothing is done very sanely here. Our real business is to get out and enter into the kingdom of God. In the *Bhagavad-gītā* Kṛṣṇa gives information of this kingdom and also gives instructions about His position and our position. All the information necessary is set forth in the *Bhagavad-gītā*, and a sane man will take advantage of this knowledge.

4
Yoga as Body and Mind Control

Throughout the *Bhagavad-gītā* Kṛṣṇa encourages Arjuna to fight, for he is a warrior and fighting is his duty. Although Kṛṣṇa delineates the meditational *yoga* system in the Sixth Chapter, He does not stress it or encourage Arjuna to pursue it as his path. Kṛṣṇa admits that this meditational process is very difficult:

śrī-bhagavān uvāca
asaṁśayaṁ mahā-bāho mano durnigrahaṁ calam
abhyāsena tu kaunteya vairāgyeṇa ca gṛhyate

"Lord Śrī Kṛṣṇa said, 'O mighty-armed son of Kuntī, it is undoubtedly very difficult to curb the restless mind, but it is possible by suitable practice and by detachment.'" (Bg. 6.35) Here Kṛṣṇa emphasizes practice and renunciation as ways to control the mind. But what is that renunciation? Today it is hardly possible for us to renounce anything, for we are so habituated to such a variety of material sense pleasures. Despite leading a life of uncontrolled sense indulgence, we attend *yoga* classes and expect to attain success. There are so many rules and regulations involved in the proper execution of *yoga,* and most of us can hardly give up a simple habit like smoking. In His discourse on the meditational *yoga* system, Kṛṣṇa proclaims that *yoga* cannot be properly performed by one who eats too much or eats too little. One who starves himself cannot properly perform *yoga.* Nor can the person who eats more than required. One should eat moderately, just enough to keep body and soul together; one should not eat for the enjoyment of the tongue. When palatable dishes come before us, we are accustomed to take not just one of the preparations but two, three, and four—and upwards. Our tongue is never satisfied. But it is not unusual in India to see a *yogī* take only a small spoonful of rice a day and nothing more. Nor can one execute the meditational *yoga* system if one sleeps too much or does not sleep sufficiently. Kṛṣṇa does not say that there is such a thing as dreamless sleep. As soon as we go to sleep, we will have a dream, although we may not remember it. In the *Gītā* Kṛṣṇa cautions that one who dreams too much while sleeping cannot properly execute *yoga*. One should not sleep more than six hours daily. Nor can one who suffers insomnia successfully execute *yoga*, for the body must be kept fit. Thus Kṛṣṇa outlines so many requirements for disciplining the body. All these requirements, however, can essentially be broken down into four basic rules: no illicit sexual connection, no intoxication, no meat-eating, and no gambling. These are the four minimum regulations for the execution of any *yoga* system. But in this age, who can refrain from these activities? We have to test ourselves accordingly to ascertain our success in *yoga* execution.

yogī yuñjīta satatam ātmānaṁ rahasi sthitaḥ
ekākī yata-cittātmā nirāśīr aparigrahaḥ

"A transcendentalist should always engage his body, mind, and self in relationship with the Supreme; he should live alone in a secluded place and should always carefully control his mind. He should be free from desires and feelings of possessiveness." (Bg. 6.10) From this verse we can understand that it is the duty of the *yogī* to always remain alone. Meditational *yoga* cannot be performed in an assembly, at least not according to the *Bhagavad-gītā*. In the meditational system it is not possible to concentrate the mind upon the Supersoul except in a secluded place. In India, there are still many *yogīs* who assemble at the Kumbha-melā. Generally they remain in seclusion, but on rare occasions they gather to attend special functions like the Kumbha-melā. Every twelve years or so thousands of *yogīs* and sages meet in particular holy places—Allahabad, etc.—just as in America they have businessmen's conventions. The *yogī*, in addition to living in a secluded place, should also be free from material desires; in other words, he should not perform *yoga* to achieve some material powers, nor should he accept gifts or favors from people. If he is properly executing meditational *yoga*, he will stay alone in the jungles, forests, or mountains and avoid society altogether. At all times he must be convinced for whom he has become a *yogī*. He does not consider himself alone because at all times the Paramātmā—Supersoul—is with him. From this we can see that in the modern civilization it is indeed very difficult to execute this meditational form of *yoga* properly. Contemporary civilization in this Age of Kali has actually made it impossible for us to be alone, to be desireless, and to be possessionless.

The method of executing meditational *yoga* is further explained in considerable detail by Kṛṣṇa to Arjuna. Śrī Kṛṣṇa says,

> *śucau deśe pratiṣṭhāpya sthiram āsanam ātmanaḥ*
> *nāty-ucchritaṁ nāti-nīcaṁ cailājina-kuśottaram*
>
> *tatraikāgraṁ manaḥ kṛtvā yata-cittendriya-kriyaḥ*
> *upaviśyāsane yuñjyād yogam ātma-viśuddhaye*

"To practice *yoga*, one should go to a secluded place and should lay *kuśa* grass on the ground and then cover it with a deerskin and a soft cloth. The seat should be neither too high nor too low and should be situated in a sacred place. The *yogī* should then sit on it very firmly and practice *yoga* to purify the heart by controlling his mind, senses, and activities and fixing the mind on one point." (Bg. 6.11–12) Generally *yogīs* sit on tiger skin or deer skin because reptiles will not crawl on such skins to disturb their meditations. It seems that in God's creation there is a use for everything. Every grass and herb has its use and serves some function, although we may not know what it is. So in the *Bhagavad-gītā* Kṛṣṇa has made some provision whereby the *yogī* doesn't have to worry about snakes. Having acquired a good sitting place in a secluded environment, the *yogī* begins to purify the *ātmā*—body, mind, and soul. The *yogī* should not think, "Now I will try to achieve some wonderful powers." Sometimes *yogīs* do attain certain *siddhis*, or mystic powers, but these are not the purpose of *yoga*, and real *yogīs* do not exhibit them. The real *yogī* thinks, "I am now contaminated by this material atmosphere, so I must purify myself."

We can quickly see that controlling the mind and body is not such an easy thing and that we cannot control them as easily as we can go to the store and purchase something. But Kṛṣṇa indicates that these rules can be easily followed when we are in Kṛṣṇa consciousness.

Of course, everyone is motivated by sex, and so in Kṛṣṇa consciousness sex is not actually discouraged. We have this material body, and as long as we have it, sex desire will be there. Similarly, as long as we have the body, we must eat to maintain it, and we must sleep in order to give it rest. We cannot expect to negate these activities, but the Vedic literatures do give us guidelines for regulation in eating, sleeping, mating, etc. If we at all expect success in *yoga*, we cannot allow our unbridled senses to take us down the paths of the sense objects; therefore guidelines are set. Lord Śrī Kṛṣṇa is advising that the mind can be controlled through regulation. If we do not regulate our activities, our mind will be more and more agitated. It is not that sensory activities are to be stopped, but they must be regulated by the mind always engaged in Kṛṣṇa consciousness. Being always engaged in some activity connected with Kṛṣṇa is actual *samādhi.* It is not that when one is in *samādhi* he doesn't eat, work, sleep, or enjoy himself in any way. Rather, *samādhi* can be defined as executing regulated activities while absorbed in thoughts of Kṛṣṇa. Such consciousness is possible with practice. As Kṛṣṇa says,

asaṁyatātmanā yogo duṣprāpa iti me matiḥ
vaśyātmanā tu yatatā śakyo 'vāptum upāyataḥ

"For one whose mind is unbridled, self-realization is difficult work. But he whose mind is controlled and who strives by right means is assured of success. That is My judgment." (Bg. 6.36) Everyone knows that an unbridled horse is dangerous to ride. He can go in any direction at any speed, and his rider is likely to come to some harm. Insofar as the mind is unbridled, Kṛṣṇa agrees with Arjuna that the *yoga* system is very difficult work indeed. "But," Kṛṣṇa adds, "he whose mind is controlled and strives by right means is assured of success. That is My judgment." (Bg. 6.36) What is meant by "strives by right means"? One has to try to follow the four basic regulative principles as mentioned and execute his activities absorbed in Kṛṣṇa consciousness.

If one wants to engage in *yoga* at home, then he has to make certain that his other engagements are moderate. He cannot spend long hours of the day working hard simply to earn a livelihood. One should work very moderately, eat very moderately, gratify the senses very moderately, and keep his life as free from anxiety as possible. In this way practice of *yoga* may be successful.

What is the sign by which we can tell that one has attained perfection in *yoga*? Kṛṣṇa indicates that one is situated in *yoga* when his consciousness is completely under his control.

yadā viniyataṁ cittam ātmany evāvatiṣṭhate
nispṛhaḥ sarva-kāmebhyo yukta ity ucyate tadā

"When the *yogī*, by practice of *yoga*, disciplines his mental activities and becomes situated in transcendence—devoid of all material desires—he is said to have attained *yoga*." (Bg. 6.18) One who has attained *yoga* is not dependent on the dictations of his mind; rather, the mind comes under his control. Nor is the mind put out or extinguished, for it is the business of the *yogī* to think of Kṛṣṇa, or Viṣṇu, always. The *yogī* cannot allow his mind to go out. This may sound very difficult, but it is possible in Kṛṣṇa consciousness. When one is always engaged in Kṛṣṇa consciousness, in the service of Kṛṣṇa, then how is it possible for the mind to wander away from Kṛṣṇa? In the service of Kṛṣṇa, the mind is automatically controlled.

Nor should the *yogī* have any desire for material sense gratification. If one is in Kṛṣṇa consciousness, he has no desire other than Kṛṣṇa. It is not possible to become desireless. The desire for sense gratification must be overcome by the process of purification, but desire for Kṛṣṇa should be cultivated. It is simply that we have to transfer the desire. There is no question of killing desire, for desire is the constant companion of the living entity. Kṛṣṇa consciousness is the process by which one purifies his desires; instead of desiring so many things for sense gratification, one simply desires things for the service of Kṛṣṇa. For example, we may desire palatable food, but instead of preparing dishes for ourselves, we can prepare them for Kṛṣṇa and offer them to Him. It is not that the action is different, but there is a transfer of consciousness from thinking and acting for my senses to thinking and acting for Kṛṣṇa. We may prepare nice milk products, vegetables, grains, fruits, and other vegetarian dishes for Kṛṣṇa and then offer them to Him, praying, "This material body is a lump of ignorance, and the senses are a network of paths leading to death. Of all the senses the tongue is the most voracious and difficult to control. It is very difficult to conquer the tongue in this world; therefore Śrī Kṛṣṇa has given us this nice *prasādam*, spiritual food, to conquer the tongue. So let us take this *prasādam* to our full satisfaction and glorify Their Lordships Śrī Śrī Rādhā and Kṛṣṇa and in love call for the help of Lord Caitanya and Nityānanda Prabhu." In this way our *karma* is neutralized, for from the very beginning we are thinking that the food is being offered to Kṛṣṇa. We should have no personal desires for the food. Kṛṣṇa is so merciful, however, that he gives us the food to eat. In this way our desire is fulfilled. When one has molded his life in such a way—dovetailing his desires to Kṛṣṇa's—then it is to be understood that he has attained perfection in *yoga*. Simply breathing deeply and doing some exercises is not *yoga* as far as the *Bhagavad-gītā* is concerned. A whole purification of consciousness is required.

In the execution of *yoga*, it is very important that the mind is not agitated.

yathā dīpo nivāta-stho neṅgate sopamā smṛtā
yogino yata-cittasya yuñjato yogam ātmanaḥ

"As a lamp in a windless place does not waver, so the transcendentalist whose mind is controlled remains always steady in his meditation on the transcendent self." (Bg. 6.19) When a candle is in a windless place, its flame remains straight and does not waver. The mind, like the flame, is susceptible to so many material desires that with the slightest agitation it will move. A little movement of the mind can change the whole consciousness. Therefore in India one who seriously practiced *yoga* traditionally remained a *brahmacārī*, a celibate. There are two kinds of *brahmacārīs:* one is completely celibate and the other is a *gṛhastha-brahmacārī*, that is to say he has a wife, he does not associate with any other woman, and his relations with his wife are strictly regulated. In this way, either by complete celibacy or by restricted sex life, one's mind is kept from being agitated. Yet when one takes a vow to remain a complete celibate, his mind may still be agitated by sexual desire; therefore in India those practicing the traditional *yoga* under strict vows of celibacy are not allowed to sit alone even with a mother, sister, or daughter. The mind is so fickle that the slightest suggestion can create havoc.

The *yogī* should train his mind in such a way that as soon as it wanders from meditation on Viṣṇu he drags it back again. This requires a great deal of practice. One must come to know that his real happiness is in experiencing the pleasure of his transcendental senses, not the material senses. The activities of the senses are not to be stopped, nor are desires to be suppressed, for there are both desires and sense satisfaction in the spiritual sphere. Real happiness is transcendental to material, sensual experience. If one is not convinced of this, he will surely be agitated and will fall down. One should therefore know that the happiness he is trying to derive from the material senses is not really happiness.

Those who are actually *yogīs* truly enjoy, but how do they enjoy? *Ramante yogino 'nante*—their enjoyment is unlimited, that unlimited enjoyment is real happiness, and such happiness is spiritual, not material. This is the real meaning of *Rāma*, as in the chant Hare Rāma. *Rāma* means enjoyment through spiritual life. Spiritual life is all pleasure, and Kṛṣṇa is all pleasure. We do not have to sacrifice pleasure, but we do have to learn how to enjoy it properly. A diseased man cannot enjoy life; his so-called enjoyment in that condition is all false enjoyment. But when he is cured and is healthy, then he is able to actually enjoy. Similarly, as long as we are in the material conception of life, we are not actually enjoying ourselves but are simply becoming more and more entangled in material nature. If a sick man is not supposed to eat, his eating unrestrictedly actually kills him. Similarly, the more we increase material enjoyment, the more we become entangled in this world, and the more difficult it becomes to get free from the material entrapment. All of the systems of *yoga* are meant to disentangle the conditioned soul from this entrapment, to transfer him from the false enjoyment of material things to the actual enjoyment of Kṛṣṇa consciousness. Śrī Kṛṣṇa says,

yatroparamate cittaṁ niruddhaṁ yoga-sevayā
yatra caivātmanātmānaṁ paśyann ātmani tuṣyati

sukham ātyantikaṁ yat tad buddhi-grāhyam atīndriyam
vetti yatra na caivāyaṁ sthitaś calati tattvataḥ

yaṁ labdhvā cāparaṁ lābhaṁ manyate nādhikaṁ tataḥ
yasmin sthito na duḥkhena guruṇāpi vicālyate

taṁ vidyād duḥkha-saṁyoga-viyogaṁ yoga-saṁjñitam

"In the stage of perfection called trance, or *samādhi*, one's mind is completely restrained from material mental activities by the practice of *yoga*. This perfection is characterized by one's ability to see the Self by the pure mind and to relish and rejoice in the Self. In that joyous state one is situated in boundless transcendental happiness, realized through transcendental senses. Established thus, one never departs from the truth, and upon gaining this he thinks there is no greater gain. Being situated in such a position, one is never shaken, even in the midst of the greatest difficulty. This indeed is actual freedom from all miseries arising from material contact." (Bg. 6.20–23) One form of *yoga* may be difficult and another may be easy, but in all cases one must purify his existence so he can experience Kṛṣṇa conscious enjoyment. Then one will be happy.

yadā hi nendriyārtheṣu na karmasv anuṣajjate
sarva-saṅkalpa-sannyāsī yogārūḍhas tadocyate

uddhared ātmanātmānaṁ nātmānam avasādayet
ātmaiva hy ātmano bandhur ātmaiva ripur ātmanaḥ

"A person is said to have attained to *yoga* when, having renounced all material desires, he neither acts for sense gratification nor engages in fruitive activities. A man must elevate himself by his own mind, not degrade himself. The mind is the friend of the conditioned soul, and his enemy as well." (Bg.

6.4–5) We have to raise ourselves to the spiritual standard by ourselves. In this sense I am my own friend and I am my own enemy. The opportunity is ours. There is a very nice verse by Cāṇakya Paṇḍita: "No one is anyone's friend, no one is anyone's enemy. It is only by behavior that one can understand who is his friend and who is his enemy." No one is born our enemy, and no one is born our friend. These roles are determined by mutual behavior. As we have dealings with others in ordinary affairs, in the same way the individual has dealings with himself. I may act as my own friend or as an enemy. As a friend, I can understand my position as a spirit soul and, seeing that somehow or other I have come into contact with material nature, try to get free from material entanglement by acting in such a way as to disentangle myself. In this case I am my friend. But if even after getting this opportunity I do not take it, then I should be considered my own worst enemy.

bandhur ātmātmanas tasya yenātmaivātmanā jitaḥ
anātmanas tu śatrutve vartetātmaiva śatru-vat

"For he who has conquered the mind, the mind is the best of friends, but for one who has failed to do so, his very mind will be the greatest enemy." (Bg. 6.6) How is it possible for one to become his own friend? This is explained here. *Ātmā* means "mind," "body," and "soul." When we are in the bodily conception and speak of *ātmā*, we refer to the body. However, when we transcend the bodily conception and rise to the mental platform, *ātmā* refers to the mind. But when we are situated on the truly spiritual platform, then *ātmā* refers to the soul. In actuality we are pure spirit. In this way, according to one's spiritual development, the meaning of the word *ātmā* differs. As far as the *Nirukti* Vedic dictionary is concerned, *ātmā* refers to the body, mind, and soul. However, in this verse of the *Bhagavad-gītā*, *ātmā* refers to the mind.

If, through *yoga*, the mind can be trained, then the mind is our friend. But if the mind is left untrained, then there is no possibility of leading a successful life. For one who has no idea of spiritual life, the mind is the enemy. If one thinks that he is simply the body, his mind will not be working for his benefit; it will simply be acting to serve the gross body and to further condition the living entity and entrap him in material nature. If, however, one understands one's position as a spirit soul apart from the body, the mind can be a liberating factor. In itself, the mind has nothing to do; it is simply waiting to be trained, and it is best trained through association. Desire is the function of the mind, and one desires according to his association; so if the mind is to act as a friend, there must be good association.

The best association is a *sādhu,* that is, a Kṛṣṇa conscious person or one who is striving for spiritual realization. There are those who are striving for temporary things (*asat*). Matter and the body are temporary, and if one only engages himself for bodily pleasure, he is conditioned by temporary things. But if he engages himself in self-realization, then he is engaged in something permanent (*sat*). Obviously if one is intelligent he will associate with those who are trying to elevate themselves to the platform of self-realization through one of the various forms of *yoga.* The result will be that those who are *sādhu,* or realized, will be able to sever his attachment to material association. This is the great advantage of good association. For instance, Kṛṣṇa speaks the *Bhagavad-gītā* to Arjuna just to cut off his attachment to this material affection. Because Arjuna is attached to things that are impeding the execution of his own duty, Kṛṣṇa severs these attachments. To cut something, a sharp instrument is required, and to cut the mind from its attachments, sharp words are often required. The *sādhu* or teacher shows no mercy in using sharp words to sever the student's mind from material attachments. By speaking the truth uncompromisingly, he is able to sever the bondage. For example, at the very beginning of the *Bhagavad-gītā* Kṛṣṇa speaks sharply to Arjuna by telling him that although he speaks like a learned man, he is actually fool number one. If we actually want detachment from this material world, we should be prepared to accept such cutting words from the spiritual master. Compromise and flattery have no effect where strong words are required.

In the *Bhagavad-gītā* the material conception of life is condemned in so many places. As an enemy is always thinking of doing harm, so the untrained mind will drag one deeper and deeper into material entanglement. Conditioned souls struggle very hard with the mind and senses. Since the mind directs the senses, it is of utmost importance to make the mind the friend.

jitātmanaḥ praśāntasya paramātmā samāhitaḥ
śītoṣṇa-sukha-duḥkheṣu tathā mānāpamānayoḥ

"For one who has conquered the mind, the Supersoul is already reached, for he has attained tranquillity. To such a man happiness and distress, heat and cold, honor and dishonor are all the same." (Bg. 6.7) By training the mind, one actually attains tranquillity, for the mind is always dragging us over impermanent things, just as an unbridled horse will pull a chariot on a perilous course. Although we are permanent and eternal, somehow or other we have become attracted to impermanent things. But the mind can be easily trained if it is simply fixed on Kṛṣṇa. Just as a fort is safe when it is defended by a great general, if Kṛṣṇa is placed in the fort of the mind, there will be no possibility of the enemy's entering. Material education, wealth, and power will not help one control the mind. A great devotee prays, "When will I be able to think of You constantly? My mind is always dragging me about, but as soon as I am able to fix my mind on the lotus feet of Kṛṣṇa, it becomes clear." When the mind is clear, it is possible to meditate on the Supersoul. The Paramātmā, or Supersoul, is always seated within the heart along with the individual soul. The *yoga* system involves concentrating the mind and focusing it on the Paramātmā, or Supersoul, seated within the heart. The previously quoted verse from the *Bhagavad-gītā* indicates that one who has conquered the mind and has overcome all attachment to impermanent things can be absorbed in thought of the Paramātmā. One so absorbed becomes free from all duality and false designations.

5

Yoga as Freedom from Duality and Designation

This material world is a world of duality—at one moment we are subjected to the heat of the summer season and at the next moment the cold of winter. Or at one moment we're happy and at the next moment distressed. At one moment honored, at the next dishonored. In the material world of duality, it is impossible to understand one thing without understanding its opposite. It is not possible to understand what honor is unless I understand dishonor. Similarly, I cannot understand what misery is if I have never tasted happiness. Nor can I understand what happiness is unless I have tasted misery. One has to transcend such dualities, but as long as this body is here these dualities will be here also. Insofar as one strives to get out of bodily conceptions—not out of the body but out of bodily conceptions—one has to learn to tolerate such dualities. In the Second Chapter of the *Bhagavad-gītā* Kṛṣṇa informs Arjuna that the duality of distress and happiness is due to the body alone. It's like a skin disease, or an itch. Just because there is an itch, one should not be mad after scratching it. We should not go mad or give up our duty just because mosquitoes bite us. There are so many dualities one has to tolerate, but if the mind is fixed in Kṛṣṇa consciousness, all these dualities will seem insignificant.

How can one tolerate such dualities?

jñāna-vijñāna-tṛptātmā kūṭa-stho vijitendriyaḥ
yukta ity ucyate yogī sama-loṣṭrāśma-kāñcanaḥ

"A person is said to be established in self-realization and is called a *yogī* (or mystic) when he is fully satisfied by virtue of acquired knowledge and realization. Such a person is situated in transcendence and is self-controlled. He sees everything—whether it be pebbles, stones, or gold—as the same." (Bg. 6.8)

Jñāna means theoretical knowledge, and *vijñāna* refers to practical knowledge. For instance, a science student has to study theoretical scientific conceptions as well as applied science. Theoretical knowledge alone will not help. One has to be able to also apply this knowledge. Similarly, in *yoga* one should have not only theoretical knowledge but practical knowledge. Simply understanding "I am not this body" and at the same time acting in a nonsensical way will not help. There are so many societies where the members seriously discuss Vedānta philosophy while smoking and drinking and enjoying a sensual life. It will not help if one only has knowledge theoretically. This knowledge must be demonstrated. One who truly understands "I am not this body" will actually reduce his bodily necessities to a minimum. When one increases the demands of the body while thinking "I am not this body," then of what use is that knowledge? A person can only be satisfied when there is *jñāna* and *vijñāna* side by aide.

When a person is situated on the practical level of spiritual realization, it should be understood that he is actually situated in *yoga.* It is not that one should continue to attend *yoga* classes and yet remain the same throughout his life; there must be practical realization. And what is the sign of that practical realization? The mind will be calm and quiet and no longer agitated by the attraction of the material world. Thus self-controlled, one is not attracted by the material glitter, and he sees everything—pebbles, stones, or gold—as the same. In the material civilization, so much paraphernalia is produced just to satisfy the senses. These things are produced under the banner of material advancement. He who is situated in *yoga* sees such paraphernalia as just so much rubbish in the street. Moreover,

suhṛn-mitrāry-udāsīna-madhyastha-dveṣya-bandhuṣu
sādhuṣv api ca pāpeṣu sama-buddhir viśiṣyate

"A person is considered still further advanced when he regards honest well-wishers, affectionate benefactors, the neutral, mediators, the envious, friends and enemies, the pious and the sinners all with an equal mind." (Bg. 6.9) There are different kinds of friends. There is *suhṛt,* who is by nature a well-wisher and is always desiring one's welfare. *Mitra* refers to an ordinary friend, and *udāsīna* is one who is neutral. In this material world someone may be my well-wisher, friend, or neither friend nor enemy but neutral. Someone else may serve as a mediator between me and my enemies, and in this verse he is called *madhya-stha.* One may also see someone as pious and another as sinful according to his own calculations. But when he is situated in transcendence, all of these—friends, enemies, or whatever—are regarded equally. When one becomes actually learned, he does not see anyone as enemy, friend, etc., for he thinks, "No one is my enemy, no one is my friend, no one is my father, no one is my mother, etc." We are all simply living entities playing on a stage in the dress of father, mother, children, friend, enemy, sinner, saint, etc. Material life is like a great drama with so many characters playing their parts. On the stage a person may be an enemy or whatever, but off the stage all the actors are friends. Similarly, with these bodies we are playing on the stage of material nature, and we attach so many designations to one another. I may be thinking, "This is my son," but in actuality I cannot beget any son. It is not possible. At the utmost I can only beget a body. It is not within any man's power to beget a living entity. Merely by sexual intercourse a living entity cannot be begotten. The living entity is simply placed in the emulsification of secretions, and a body develops around him. This is the verdict of *Śrīmad-Bhāgavatam.* Thus all the multifarious relationships between bodies are just so much stage play. One who is actually realized and has actually attained *yoga* no longer sees these bodily distinctions.

6

The Fate of the Unsuccessful Yogī

It is not that the *Bhagavad-gītā* rejects the meditational *yoga* process; it recognizes it as a bona fide method, but it further indicates that it is not possible in this age. Thus in the Sixth Chapter of the *Bhagavad-gītā* the subject of meditation is quickly dropped by Śrī Kṛṣṇa and Arjuna. Arjuna next asks,

ayatiḥ śraddhayopeto yogāc calita-mānasaḥ
aprāpya yoga-saṁsiddhiṁ kāṁ gatiṁ kṛṣṇa gacchati

"O Kṛṣṇa, what is the destination of the unsuccessful transcendentalist, who in the beginning takes to the process of self-realization with faith but who later desists due to worldly-mindedness and thus does not attain perfection in mysticism?" (Bg. 6.37) In other words, he is asking what becomes of the unsuccessful *yogī*, or the person who attempts to perform *yoga* but somehow desists and does not succeed. Such a *yogī* is something like a student who does not get his degree because he drops out of school. Elsewhere in the *Gītā*, Śrī Kṛṣṇa points out to Arjuna that out of many men, few strive for perfection, and out of those who strive for perfection, only a few succeed. So Arjuna is inquiring after the vast number of failures. Even if a man has faith and strives for perfection in the *yoga* system, Arjuna points out that he may not attain this perfection due to worldly-mindedness.

kaccin nobhaya-vibhraṣṭaś chinnābhram iva naśyati
apratiṣṭho mahā-bāho vimūḍho brahmaṇaḥ pathi

"O mighty-armed Kṛṣṇa," Arjuna continues, "does not such a man, who out of bewilderment deviates from the path of transcendence, fall away from both spiritual and material success and perish like a riven cloud, with no position in any sphere?" (Bg. 6.38) When a cloud is torn apart by the wind, it does not mend back together again.

etan me saṁśayaṁ kṛṣṇa chettum arhasy aśeṣataḥ
tvad-anyaḥ saṁśayasyāsya chettā na hy upapadyate

"This is my doubt, O Kṛṣṇa, and I ask You to dispel it completely. But for You, no one is to be found who can destroy this doubt." (Bg. 6.39) Arjuna is asking this question about the fate of the unsuccessful *yogī* so that in the future people would not be discouraged. By a *yogī,* Arjuna is referring not only to the *dhyāna-yogī* but also to the *karma-yogī, jñāna-yogī,* and *bhakti-yogī;* it is not that meditation is the only form of *yoga.* The renounced worker, the meditator, the philosopher, and the devotee are all to be considered *yogīs.* Arjuna is questioning for all those who are attempting to become successful transcendentalists. And how does Śrī Kṛṣṇa answer him?

śrī-bhagavān uvāca
pārtha naiveha nāmutra vināśas tasya vidyate
na hi kalyāṇa-kṛt kaścid durgatiṁ tāta gacchati

Here, as in many other places throughout the *Gītā,* Śrī Kṛṣṇa is referred to as Bhagavān. This is another of the Lord's innumerable names. *Bhagavān* indicates that Kṛṣṇa is the proprietor of six opulences: He possesses all beauty, all wealth, all power, all fame, all knowledge, and all renunciation. Living entities partake of these opulences in finite degrees. One may be famous in a family, in a town, in a country, or on one planet, but no one is famous throughout the creation, as is Śrī Kṛṣṇa. The leaders of the world may be famous for a few years only, but Lord Śrī Kṛṣṇa appeared five thousand years ago and is still being worshiped. So one who possesses all six of these opulences in completeness is considered to be God. In the *Bhagavad-gītā* Kṛṣṇa speaks to Arjuna as the Supreme Personality of Godhead, and as such it is to be understood that He has complete knowledge. The *Bhagavad-gītā* was imparted to the sun-god and to Arjuna by Kṛṣṇa, but nowhere is it mentioned that the *Bhagavad-gītā* was imparted to Kṛṣṇa. Why? Complete knowledge means that He knows everything that is to be known. This is an attribute of God alone. Being that Kṛṣṇa knows everything, Arjuna is putting this question to Him about the fate of the unsuccessful *yogī.* There is no possibility for Arjuna to research the truth. He simply has to receive the truth from the complete source, and this is the system of disciplic succession. Kṛṣṇa is complete, and the knowledge that comes from Kṛṣṇa is also complete. If Arjuna receives this complete knowledge and we receive it from Arjuna as it was spoken to him, then we also receive complete knowledge. And what is this knowledge? "Lord Kṛṣṇa said, O son of Pṛthā, a transcendentalist engaged in auspicious activities does not meet with destruction either in this world or in the spiritual world; one who does good, My friend, is never overcome by evil." (Bg. 6.40) Here Kṛṣṇa indicates that the very striving for perfection in *yoga* is a most auspicious attempt. When one attempts something so auspicious, he is never degraded.

Actually Arjuna is asking a very appropriate and intelligent question. It is not unusual for one to fall down from the platform of devotional service. Sometimes a neophyte devotee does not keep the rules and regulations. Sometimes he yields to intoxication or is trapped by some feminine attractions. These are impediments on the path of *yoga* perfection. But Śrī Kṛṣṇa gives an encouraging answer, for He tells Arjuna that even if one sincerely cultivates only one-percent worth of spiritual knowledge, he will never fall down into the material whirlpool. That is due to the sincerity of his effort. It should always be understood that we are weak and that the material energy is very strong. To adopt spiritual life is more or less to declare war against the material energy. The material energy is trying to entrap the conditioned soul as much as possible, and when the conditioned soul tries to get out of her clutches by spiritual advancement of knowledge, the material nature becomes more stringent and vigorous in her efforts to test how much the aspiring spiritualist is sincere. The material energy, or *māyā*, will then offer more allurements.

In this regard there is the story of Viśvāmitra Muni, a great king, a *kṣatriya*, who renounced his kingdom and took to the *yoga* process in order to become spiritually advanced. At that time the meditational *yoga* process was possible to execute. Viśvāmitra Muni meditated so intently that Indra, the King of heaven, noticed him and thought, "This man is trying to occupy my post." The heavenly planets are also material, and there is competition—no businessman wants another businessman to excel him. Fearing that Viśvāmitra Muni would actually depose him, Indra sent a heavenly society girl named Menakā to allure him sexually. Menakā was naturally very beautiful, and she was intent on disrupting the *muni's* meditations. Indeed, he became aware of her feminine presence upon hearing the sound of her ankle bells, and he immediately looked up from his meditation, saw her, and became captivated by her beauty. As a result, the beautiful girl Śakuntalā was born by their conjugation. When Śakuntalā was born, Viśvāmitra lamented, "Oh, I was just trying to cultivate spiritual knowledge, and again I have been entrapped." He was about to flee when Menakā brought his beautiful daughter before him and chastised him. Despite her pleading, Viśvāmitra resolved to leave anyway.

Thus there is every chance of failure on the yogic path; even a great sage like Viśvāmitra Muni can fall down due to material allurement. Although the *muni* fell for the time being, he again resolved to go on with the *yoga* process, and this should be our resolve. Kṛṣṇa informs us that such failures should not be a cause for despair. There is the famous proverb that "failure is the pillar of success." In the spiritual life especially, failure is not discouraging. Kṛṣṇa very clearly states that even if there is failure, there is no loss either in this world or in the next. One who takes to this auspicious line of spiritual culture is never completely vanquished.

Now what actually happens to the unsuccessful spiritualist? Śrī Kṛṣṇa specifically explains,

prāpya puṇya-kṛtāṁ lokān uṣitvā śāśvatīḥ samāḥ
śucīnāṁ śrīmatāṁ gehe yoga-bhraṣṭo 'bhijāyate

athavā yoginām eva kule bhavati dhīmatām
etad dhi durlabhataraṁ loke janma yad īdṛśam

"The unsuccessful *yogī*, after many, many years of enjoyment on the planets of the pious living entities, is born into a family of righteous people, or into a family of rich aristocracy. Or he takes his birth in a family of transcendentalists who are surely great in wisdom. Verily, such a birth is rare in this world." (Bg. 6.41–42) There are many planets in the universe, and on the higher planets there are greater comforts, the duration of life is longer, and the inhabitants are more religious and godly. Since it is said that a period of six months on earth is equal to one day on the higher planets, the unsuccessful *yogī* stays on these higher planets for many, many years. The Vedic literatures describe the lifetimes of the residents of heaven as lasting ten thousand years. So even if one is a failure, he is promoted to these higher planets. But one cannot remain there perpetually. When the results of one's pious activities expire, he has to return to earth. Yet even upon returning to this planet, the unsuccessful *yogī* meets with fortunate circumstances, for he takes his birth in either a very rich family or a pious one.

Generally, according to the law of *karma,* one who performs pious deeds is rewarded in the next life with birth into a very aristocratic or wealthy family, or he becomes a great scholar, or he is born very beautiful. In any case, those who sincerely begin spiritual life are guaranteed a human birth in the next life—not only a human birth, but birth into either a very pious or wealthy family. Thus one with such a good birth should understand that his fortune is due to his previous pious activities and to God's grace. These facilities are given by the Lord, who is always willing to give us the means to attain Him. Kṛṣṇa simply wants to see that we are sincere. In *Śrīmad-Bhāgavatam* it is stated that every person has his own duty in life, regardless of his position and regardless of his society. If, however, he gives up his prescribed duty and somehow or other takes shelter of Kṛṣṇa—either out of sentiment or association or craziness or whatever—and if, due to his immaturity, he falls from the devotional path, still there is no loss for him. On the other hand, if a person executes his duties perfectly but does not approach God, then what does he earn? His life is indeed without benefit. But a person who has approached Kṛṣṇa is better situated, even though he may fall down from the yogic platform.

Kṛṣṇa further indicates that of all good families to be born into—families of successful merchants or philosophers or meditators—the best is the family of *yogīs.* One who takes birth in a very rich family may be misled. It is normal for a man who is given great riches to try to enjoy those riches; thus rich men's sons often become drunkards or prostitute hunters. Similarly, one who takes birth in a pious family or in a brahminical family often becomes very puffed up and proud, thinking, "I am a *brāhmaṇa;* I am a pious man." There is a chance of degradation in both rich and pious families, but one who takes birth in a family of *yogīs* or devotees has a much better chance of again cultivating that spiritual life from which he has fallen. Kṛṣṇa tells Arjuna,

tatra taṁ buddhi-saṁyogaṁ labhate paurva-dehikam
yatate ca tato bhūyaḥ saṁsiddhau kuru-nandana

"On taking such a birth he revives the divine consciousness of his previous life, and he tries to make further progress in order to achieve complete success, O son of Kuru." (Bg. 6.43)

Being born in a family of those who execute *yoga* or devotional service, one remembers his spiritual activities executed in his previous life. Anyone who takes to Kṛṣṇa consciousness seriously is not an ordinary person; he must have taken to the same process in his previous life. Why is this?

pūrvābhyāsena tenaiva hriyate hy avaśo 'pi saḥ

"By virtue of the divine consciousness of his previous life, he automatically becomes attracted to the yogic principles—even without seeking them." (Bg. 6.44) In the material world we have experience that we do not carry our assets from one life to another. I may have millions of dollars in the bank, but as soon as my body is finished, my relationship with my bank balance is also finished. At death, the bank balance does not go with me; it remains in the bank to be enjoyed by somebody else. This is not the case with spiritual culture. Even if one enacts a very small amount on the spiritual platform, he takes that with him to his next life, and he picks up again from that point.

When one picks up this knowledge that was interrupted, he should know that he should now finish the balance and complete the yogic process. One should not take the chance of finishing up the process in another birth but should resolve to finish it in this life. We should be determined in this way: "Somehow or other in my last life I did not finish my spiritual cultivation. Now Kṛṣṇa has given me another opportunity, so let me finish it up in this life." Thus after leaving this body one will not again take birth in this material world, where birth, old age, disease, and death are omnipresent, but will return to Kṛṣṇa. One who takes shelter under the lotus feet of Kṛṣṇa sees this material world simply as a place of danger. For one who takes to spiritual culture, this material world is actually unfit. Śrīla Bhaktisiddhānta Sarasvatī used to say, "This place is not fit for a gentleman." Once one has approached Kṛṣṇa and has attempted to make spiritual progress, Kṛṣṇa, who is situated within the heart, begins to give directions. In the *Gītā* Śrī Kṛṣṇa says that for one who wants to remember Him, He gives remembrance, and for one who wants to forget Him, He allows him to forget.

7
Yoga as Reestablishing One's Relationship with Kṛṣṇa

The aim of the *yoga* system Kṛṣṇa describes in the *Bhagavad-gītā* is threefold: to control the senses, to purify activities, and to link oneself to Kṛṣṇa in a reciprocal relationship.

The Absolute Truth is realized in three stages: impersonal Brahman, localized Paramātmā (Supersoul), and ultimately Bhagavān, the Supreme Personality of Godhead. In the final analysis, the Supreme Absolute Truth is a person. Simultaneously He is the all-pervading Supersoul within the hearts of all living entities and within the core of all atoms, and He is the *brahmajyoti*, or the effulgence of spiritual light, as well. Bhagavān Śrī Kṛṣṇa, being the Supreme Personality of Godhead, is full in all opulences, but at the same time He is fully renounced. In the material world we find that one who has much opulence is not very much inclined to give it up, but Kṛṣṇa is not like this. He can renounce everything and remain complete in Himself.

When we study the *Bhagavad-gītā* under a bona fide spiritual master, we should not think that the spiritual master is presenting his own opinions. It is not he who is speaking. He is just an instrument. The real speaker is the Supreme Personality of Godhead, who is both within and without. At the beginning of His discourse on the *yoga* system in the Sixth Chapter of the *Bhagavad-gītā*, Śrī Kṛṣṇa says,

anāśritaḥ karma-phalaṁ kāryaṁ karma karoti yaḥ
sa sannyāsī ca yogī ca na niragnir na cākriyaḥ

"One who is unattached to the fruits of his work and who works as he is obligated is in the renounced order of life, and he is the true mystic; not he who lights no fire and performs no work." (Bg. 6.1) Everyone is working and expecting some result. One may ask, What is the purpose of working if no result is expected? A remuneration or salary is always demanded by the worker. But here Kṛṣṇa indicates that one can work out of a sense of duty alone, not expecting the results of his activities. If one works in this way, then he is actually a *sannyāsī;* he is in the renounced order of life.

According to the Vedic culture, there are four stages of life: *brahmacarya, gṛhastha, vānaprastha,* and *sannyāsa. Brahmacarya* is student life devoted to training in spiritual understanding. *Gṛhastha* life is married householder life. Then upon reaching the approximate age of fifty, one may take the *vānaprastha* order—that is, he leaves his home and children and travels with his wife to holy places of pilgrimage. Finally he gives up both wife and children and remains alone to cultivate Kṛṣṇa consciousness, and that stage is called *sannyāsa,* or the renounced order of life. Yet Kṛṣṇa indicates that for a *sannyāsī,* renunciation is not all. In addition, there must be some duty. What then is the duty for a *sannyāsī,* for one who has renounced family life and no longer has material obligations? His duty is a most responsible one: to work for Kṛṣṇa. Moreover, this is the real duty for everyone in all stages of life.

In everyone's life there are two duties: one is to serve the illusion, and the other is to serve the reality. When one serves the reality, he is a real *sannyāsī.* And when one serves the illusion, he is deluded by *māyā.* One has to understand, however, that he is in all circumstances forced to serve. Either he serves the illusion or the reality. The constitutional position of the living entity is to be a servant, not a master. One may think that he is the master, but he is actually a servant. When one has a family he may think that he is the master of his wife, children, home, business, and so on, but that is all false. One is actually the servant of his wife, children, and so on. The president may be considered the master of the country, but actually he is the servant of the country. Our position is always as servant—either as servant of the illusion or as servant of God. If, however, we remain the servant of the illusion, then our life is wasted. Of course, everyone is thinking that he is not a servant, that he is working only for himself. Although the fruits of his labor are transient and illusory, they force him to become a servant of illusion, or a servant of his own senses. But when one awakens to his transcendental senses and actually becomes situated in knowledge, he becomes a servant of the reality. When one comes to the platform of knowledge, he understands that in all circumstances he is a servant. Since it is not possible for him to be a master, he is much better situated serving the reality instead of the illusion. When one becomes aware of this, he attains the platform of real knowledge. By *sannyāsa,* the renounced order of life, we refer to one who has come to this platform. *Sannyāsa* is a question of realization, not social status.

It is the duty of everyone to become Kṛṣṇa conscious and to serve the cause of Kṛṣṇa. When one actually realizes this he becomes a *mahātmā,* or a great soul. In the *Bhagavad-gītā* Kṛṣṇa says that after many births, when one comes to the platform of real knowledge, he surrenders unto Kṛṣṇa. Why is this? *Vāsudevaḥ sarvam iti.* The wise man realizes that Vāsudeva (Kṛṣṇa) is everything. However, Kṛṣṇa says that such a great soul is rarely found. Why is this? If an intelligent person comes to understand that the ultimate goal of life is to surrender unto Kṛṣṇa, why should he hesitate? Why not surrender immediately? What is the point in waiting for so many births? When one comes to that point of surrender, he becomes a real *sannyāsī.* Kṛṣṇa never forces anyone to surrender unto Him. Surrender is a result of love, transcendental love, and that love must be freely given. Where there is force, there can be no love. When a mother loves a child, she is not forced to do so, nor does she do so out of expectation of some salary or remuneration.

Similarly, we can love the Supreme Lord in so many ways—we can love Him as master, as friend, as child, or as husband. There are five basic *rasas,* or relationships, in which we are eternally related to God. When we are actually in the liberated stage of knowledge, we can understand that our relationship with the Lord is in a particular *rasa.* That platform is called *svarūpa-siddhi,* or real self-realization. Everyone has an eternal relationship with the Lord, either as master and servant, friend and friend, child and parent, husband and wife, or lover and beloved. These relationships are eternally present. The whole process of spiritual realization and the actual perfection of *yoga* is to revive our consciousness of this relationship. At present our relationship with the Supreme Lord is pervertedly reflected in this material world. In the material world, the relationship between master and servant is based on money or force or exploitation. There is no question of service out of love. The relationship between master and servant, pervertedly reflected, continues only for as long as the master can pay the servant. As soon as the payment stops, the relationship also stops. Similarly, in the material world there may be a relationship between friends, but as soon as there is a slight disagreement, the friendship breaks, and the friend becomes an enemy. When there is a difference of opinion between son and parents, the son leaves home and the relationship is severed. The same with husband and wife: a slight difference of opinion, and there is divorce.

No relationship in this material world is eternal. We must always remember that these ephemeral relationships are simply perverted reflections of that eternal relationship we have with the Supreme Personality of Godhead. We have experience that the reflection of an object in a glass is not real. It may appear real, but when we go to touch it we find that there is only glass. We must come to understand that these relationships as friend, parent, child, master, servant, husband, wife, or lover are simply reflections of the relationship we have with God. When we come to this platform of understanding, then we are perfect in knowledge. When that knowledge comes, we begin to understand that we are servants of Kṛṣṇa and that we have an eternal loving relationship with Him.

In this loving relationship there is no question of remuneration, but of course remuneration is there, and it is much greater than whatever we earn here through the rendering of service. There is no limit to Śrī Kṛṣṇa's remuneration. In this connection there is the story of Bali Mahārāja, a very powerful king who conquered the heavenly planets. The denizens of heaven appealed to the Supreme Lord to save them, for they had been conquered by the demoniac king, Bali Mahārāja. Upon hearing their pleas, Śrī Kṛṣṇa took the shape of a dwarf *brāhmaṇa* boy and approached Bali Mahārāja, saying, "My dear king, I would like something from you. You are a great monarch and are renowned for giving charity to the *brāhmaṇas*, so would you give Me something?"

Bali Mahārāja said, "I will give You whatever You want."

"I simply want whatever land I can cover in three steps," the boy said.

"Oh, is that all?" the king replied. "And what will You do with such a small piece of land?"

"Though it may be small, it will satisfy Me," the boy smiled.

Bali Mahārāja agreed, and the boy-dwarf took two steps and covered the entire universe. He then asked Bali Mahārāja where He was going to take His third step, and Bali Mahārāja, understanding that the Supreme Lord was showing him His favor, replied, "My dear Lord, I have now lost everything. I have no other property, but I do have my head. Would You so kindly step there?"

Lord Śrī Kṛṣṇa was then very much pleased with Bali Mahārāja, and He asked, "What would you like from Me?"

"I never expected anything from You," Bali Mahārāja said. "But I understand that You wanted something from me, and now I have offered You everything."

"Yes," the Lord said, "but from My side I have something for you. I shall always remain as an order-carrier servant in your court." In this way the Lord became Bali Mahārāja's doorman, and that was his return. If we offer something to the Lord, it is returned millions of times. But we should not expect this. The Lord is always eager to return the service of His servant. Whoever thinks that serving the Lord is actually his duty is perfect in knowledge and has attained the perfection of *yoga.*

8
The Perfection of Yoga

In the progress of the living entity toward the perfection of *yoga*, birth in a family of *yogīs* or devotees is a great boon, for such a birth gives one special impetus.

prayatnād yatamānas tu yogī saṁśuddha-kilbiṣaḥ
aneka-janma-saṁsiddhas tato yāti parāṁ gatim

"And when the *yogī* engages himself with sincere endeavor in making further progress, being washed of all contaminations, then ultimately, achieving perfection after many, many births of practice, he attains the supreme goal." (Bg. 6.45) When one is finally freed from all contaminations, he attains the supreme perfection of the *yoga* system—Kṛṣṇa consciousness. Absorption in Kṛṣṇa is the perfect stage, as Kṛṣṇa Himself confirms:

bahūnāṁ janmanām ante jñānavān māṁ prapadyate
vāsudevaḥ sarvam iti sa mahātmā sudurlabhaḥ

"After many births and deaths, he who is actually in knowledge surrenders unto Me, knowing Me to be the cause of all causes and all that is. Such a great soul is very rare." (Bg. 7.19) Thus after many lifetimes of executing pious activities, when one becomes freed from all contaminations arising from illusory dualities, he engages in the transcendental service of the Lord. Śrī Kṛṣṇa concludes His discourse on this subject in this way:

yoginām api sarveṣāṁ mad-gatenāntarātmanā
śraddhāvān bhajate yo māṁ sa me yuktatamo mataḥ

"And of all *yogīs*, the one with great faith who always abides in Me, thinks of Me within himself, and renders transcendental loving service to Me—he is the most intimately united with

Me in *yoga* and is the highest of all. That is My opinion." (Bg. 6.47) It therefore follows that the culmination of all *yogas* lies in *bhakti-yoga*, the rendering of devotional service unto Kṛṣṇa. Actually, all the *yogas* delineated in the *Bhagavad-gītā* end on this note, for Kṛṣṇa is the ultimate destination of all the *yoga* systems. From the beginning of *karma-yoga* to the end of *bhakti-yoga* is a long way to self-realization. *Karma-yoga*, in which one works without desiring fruitive results, is the beginning of this path. When *karma-yoga* increases in knowledge and renunciation, the stage is called *jñāna-yoga*, or the *yoga* of knowledge. When *jñāna-yoga* increases in meditation on the Supersoul by different physical processes and the mind is on Him, it is called *aṣṭāṅga-yoga*. And when one surpasses *aṣṭāṅga-yoga* and comes to the point of worshiping the Supreme Personality of Godhead, Kṛṣṇa, that is called *bhakti-yoga*, the culmination. Factually, *bhakti-yoga* is the ultimate goal, but to analyze *bhakti-yoga* minutely one has to understand the other processes. The *yogī* who is progressive is therefore on the true path to eternal good fortune. One who sticks to a particular point and does not make further progress is called by that particular name—*karma-yogī*, *jñāna-yogī*, *dhyāna-yogī*, *rāja-yogī*, *haṭha-yogī*, etc.—but if one is fortunate enough to come to the point of *bhakti-yoga*, Kṛṣṇa consciousness, it is to be understood that he has surpassed all the other *yoga* systems.

Kṛṣṇa consciousness is the last link in the yogic chain, the link that binds us to the Supreme Person, Lord Śrī Kṛṣṇa. Without this final link, the chain is useless. One who is truly interested in the perfection of *yoga* should immediately take to Kṛṣṇa consciousness by chanting the Hare Kṛṣṇa *mantra*, studying the *Bhagavad-gītā*, and rendering service to Kṛṣṇa through the International Society for Krishna Consciousness. In this way one will surpass all other *yoga* systems and attain the ultimate goal of all *yoga*—love for Kṛṣṇa.

Appendixes

The Author

His Divine Grace A. C. Bhaktivedanta Swami Prabhupāda appeared in this world in 1896 in Calcutta, India. He first met his spiritual master, Śrīla Bhaktisiddhānta Sarasvatī Gosvāmī, in Calcutta in 1922. Bhaktisiddhānta Sarasvatī, a prominent religious scholar and the founder of sixty-four Gauḍīya Maṭhas (Vedic institutes), liked this educated young man and convinced him to dedicate his life to teaching Vedic knowledge. Śrīla Prabhupāda became his student and, in 1933, his formally initiated disciple.

At their first meeting, in 1922, Śrīla Bhaktisiddhānta Sarasvatī requested Śrīla Prabhupāda to broadcast Vedic knowledge in English. In the years that followed, Śrīla Prabhupāda wrote a commentary on the *Bhagavad-gītā,* assisted the Gauḍīya Maṭha in its work, and, in 1944, started *Back to Godhead,* an English fortnightly magazine. Maintaining the publication was a struggle. Single-handedly Śrīla Prabhupāda edited it, typed the manuscripts, checked the galley proofs, and even distributed the individual copies. The magazine is now being continued by his disciples.

Recognizing Śrīla Prabhupāda's deep devotion and erudition, the Gauḍīya Vaiṣṇava society honored him in 1947 with the title "Bhaktivedānta," meaning "one who embodies devotion to Kṛṣṇa as the culmination of all knowledge." In 1950, at the age of fifty-four, Śrīla Prabhupāda retired from married life, adopting the *vānaprastha* (retired) order to devote more time to his studies and writing. He traveled to the holy city of Vṛndāvana, near Delhi, where he lived in humble circumstances in the historic temple of Rādhā-Dāmodara. There he engaged for several years in deep study and writing. He accepted the renounced order of life (*sannyāsa*) in 1959. At Rādhā-Dāmodara, Śrīla Prabhupāda began work on his life's masterpiece: a multivolume commentated translation of the eighteen-thousand-verse *Śrīmad-Bhāgavatam* (*Bhāgavata Purāṇa*). He also wrote *Easy Journey to Other Planets.*

After publishing three volumes of the *Bhāgavatam*, in 1965 Śrīla Prabhupāda traveled by ship to the United States to fulfill the mission of his spiritual master. Subsequently His Divine Grace wrote more than fifty volumes of authoritative commentated translations and summary studies of the philosophical and religious classics of India.

When he first arrived by freighter in New York City in September of 1965, Śrīla Prabhupāda was practically penniless. Only after almost a year of great difficulty did he succeed in establishing the International Society for Krishna Consciousness, in July of 1966. Before he passed away on November 14, 1977, he had guided the Society and seen it grow to a worldwide confederation of more than one hundred *āśramas*, schools, temples, institutes, and farm communities.

In 1968 Śrīla Prabhupāda created New Vrindaban, a rural Vedic community in the hills of West Virginia. Inspired by the success of New Vrindaban, now a thriving farm community of more than two thousand acres, his students have founded several similar communities in the United States and around the world.

In 1972 His Divine Grace introduced the Vedic system of primary and secondary education in the West by founding the *gurukula* school in Dallas, Texas. Since then his disciples have established similar schools throughout the world.

Śrīla Prabhupāda also inspired the construction of several large international cultural centers in India. The center at Śrīdhāma Māyāpur, in West Bengal, is the site for a planned spiritual city, an ambitions project for which construction will continue for many years to come. In Vṛndāvana are the magnificent Kṛṣṇa-Balarāma Temple and International Guesthouse, *gurukula* school, and Śrīla Prabhupāda Memorial and Museum. There are also major temples and cultural centers in Mumbai, New Delhi, and Bangalore. Other centers are planned in a dozen important locations on the Indian subcontinent.

Śrīla Prabhupāda's most significant contribution, however, is his books. Highly respected by scholars for their authority, depth, and clarity, they are used as textbooks in numerous college courses. His writings have been translated into over fifty languages. The Bhaktivedanta Book Trust, established in 1972 to publish the works of His Divine Grace, has thus become the world's largest publisher of books in the field of Indian religion and philosophy.

In just twelve years, in spite of his advanced age, Śrīla Prabhupāda circled the globe fourteen times on lecture tours that took him to six continents. In spite of such a vigorous schedule, he continued to write prolifically. His writings constitute a veritable library of Vedic philosophy, religion, literature, and culture.

What Is the International Society for Krishna Consciousness?

The International Society for Krishna Consciousness (ISKCON), popularly known as the Hare Kṛṣṇa movement, is a worldwide association of devotees of Kṛṣṇa, the Supreme Personality of Godhead. God is known by many names, according to His different qualities and activities. In the Bible he is known as Jehovah ("the almighty one"), in the Koran as Allah ("the great one"), and in the *Bhagavad-gītā* as Kṛṣṇa, a Sanskrit name meaning "the all-attractive one."

The movement's main purpose is to promote the well-being of human society by teaching the science of God consciousness (Kṛṣṇa consciousness) according to the timeless Vedic scriptures of India.

Many leading figures in the international religious and academic community have affirmed the movement's authenticity. Diana L. Eck, professor of comparative religion and Indian studies at Harvard University, describes the movement as a "tradition that commands a respected place in the religious life of humankind."

In 1965, His Divine Grace A. C. Bhaktivedanta Swami, known to his followers as Śrīla Prabhupāda, brought Kṛṣṇa consciousness to America. On the day he landed in Boston, on his way to New York City, he penned these words in his diary: "My dear Lord Kṛṣṇa, I am sure that when this transcendental message penetrates [the hearts of the Westerners], they will certainly feel gladdened and thus become liberated from all unhappy conditions of life." He was sixty-nine years old, alone and with few resources, but the wealth of spiritual knowledge and devotion he possessed was an unwavering source of strength and inspiration.

"At a very advanced age, when most people would be resting on their laurels," writes Harvey Cox, Harvard University theologian and author, "Śrīla Prabhupāda harkened to the mandate of his own spiritual teacher and set out on the difficult and demanding voyage to America. Śrīla Prabhupāda is, of course, only one of thousands of teachers. But in another sense, he is one in a thousand, maybe one in a million."

In 1966, Śrīla Prabhupāda founded the International Society for Krishna Consciousness, which became the formal name for the Hare Kṛṣṇa movement.

Astonishing Growth

In the years that followed, Śrīla Prabhupāda gradually attracted tens of thousands of followers, started more than a hundred temples and ashrams, and published scores of books. His achievement is remarkable in that he transplanted India's ancient spiritual culture to the twentieth-century Western world.

New devotees of Kṛṣṇa soon became highly visible in all the major cities around the world through their public chanting and their distribution of Śrīla Prabhupāda's books of Vedic knowledge. They began staging joyous cultural festivals throughout the year and serving millions of plates of delicious vegetarian food offered to Kṛṣṇa (known as *prasādam*). As a result, ISKCON has significantly influenced the lives of millions of people. In the early 1980's the late A. L. Basham, one of the world's leading authorities on Indian history and culture, wrote, "The Hare Kṛṣṇa movement arose out of next to nothing in less than twenty years and has become known all over the West. This is an important fact in the history of the Western world."

Five Thousand Years of Spiritual Wisdom

Scholars worldwide have acclaimed Śrīla Prabhupāda's translations of Vedic literature. Garry Gelade, a professor at Oxford University's Department of Philosophy, wrote of them: "These texts are to be treasured. No one of whatever faith or philosophical persuasion who reads these books with an open mind can fail to be moved and impressed." And Dr. Larry Shinn, Dean of the College of Arts and Sciences at Bucknell University, wrote, "Prabhupāda's personal piety gave him real authority. He exhibited complete command of the scriptures, an unusual depth of realization, and an outstanding personal example, because he actually lived what he taught."

The best known of the Vedic texts, the *Bhagavad-gītā* ("Song of God"), is the philosophical basis for the Hare Kṛṣṇa movement. Dating back 5,000 years, it is sacred to nearly a billion people today. This exalted work has been praised by scholars and leaders the world over. Mahatma Gandhi said, "When doubts haunt me, when disappointments stare me in the face and I see not one ray of hope, I turn to the *Bhagavad-gītā* and find a verse to comfort me." Ralph Waldo Emerson wrote, "It was the first of books; it was as if an empire spoke to us, nothing small or unworthy, but large, serene, consistent, the voice of an old intelligence which in another age and climate had pondered and thus disposed of the same questions which exercise us." It is not surprising to anyone familiar with the *Gītā* that Henry David Thoreau said, "In the morning I bathe my intellect in the stupendous and cosmogonal philosophy of the *Bhagavad-gītā*."

As Dr. Shinn pointed out, Śrīla Prabhupāda's *Bhagavad-gītā* (titled *Bhagavad-gītā As It Is*) possesses unique authority not only because of his erudition but because he lived what he taught. Thus unlike the many other English translations of the *Gītā* that preceded his, which is replete with extensive commentary, Śrīla Prabhupāda's has sparked a spiritual revolution throughout the world.

Lord Kṛṣṇa teaches in the *Bhagavad-gītā* that we are not these temporary material bodies but spirit souls, or conscious entities, and that we can find genuine peace and happiness only in spiritual devotion to God. The *Gītā* and other well-known world scriptures recommend that people joyfully chant God's holy names, such as Kṛṣṇa, Allah, and Jehovah.

A Sixteenth-Century Incarnation of Kṛṣṇa

Lord Śrī Caitanya Mahāprabhu, a sixteenth-century full incarnation of Kṛṣṇa, popularized the chanting of God's names all over India. He constantly sang these names of God, as prescribed in the Vedic literatures: Hare Kṛṣṇa, Hare Kṛṣṇa, Kṛṣṇa Kṛṣṇa, Hare Hare/ Hare Rāma, Hare Rāma, Rāma Rāma, Hare Hare. This Hare Kṛṣṇa chant, or *mantra,* is a transcendental sound vibration. It purifies the mind and awakens the dormant love of God that resides in the hearts of all living beings. Lord Caitanya requested His followers to spread the chanting to every town and village of the world.

Anyone can take part in the chanting of the Hare Kṛṣṇa *mantra* and learn the science of spiritual devotion by studying the *Bhagavad-gītā As It Is.* This easy and practical process of self-realization will awaken our natural state of peace and happiness.

Hare Kṛṣṇa Lifestyles

The devotees seen dancing and chanting in the streets, dressed in traditional Indian robes, are for the most part full-time students of the Hare Kṛṣṇa movement. The vast majority of followers, however, live and work in the general community, practicing Kṛṣṇa consciousness in their homes and attending temples on a regular basis.

Full-time devotees throughout the world number about 15,000, with 500,000 congregational members. The movement comprises 300 temples, 50 rural communities, 40 schools, and 75 restaurants in 85 countries.

In order to revive their own and humanity's inherent natural spiritual principles of compassion, truthfulness, cleanliness, and austerity, and to master the mind and the material senses, devotees also follow these four regulations:

1. No eating of meat, fish, or eggs.
2. No gambling.
3. No illicit sex.
4. No intoxication of any kind, including tobacco, coffee, and tea.

According to the *Bhagavad-gītā* and other Vedic literatures, indulgence in the above activities disrupts our physical, mental, and spiritual well-being and increases anxiety and conflict in society.

A Philosophy for Everyone

The philosophy of the Hare Kṛṣṇa movement (a monotheistic tradition) is summarized in the following eight points:

1. By sincerely cultivating the authentic spiritual science presented in the *Bhagavad-gītā* and other Vedic scriptures, we can become free from anxiety and achieve a state of pure, unending, blissful consciousness.
2. Each of us is not the material body but an eternal spirit soul, part and parcel of God (Kṛṣṇa). As such, we are all the

eternal servants of Kṛṣṇa and are interrelated through Him, our common father.

3. Kṛṣṇa is the eternal, all-knowing, omnipresent, all-powerful, and all-attractive Personality of Godhead. He is the seed-giving father of all living beings and the sustaining energy of the universe. He is the source of all incarnations of God, including Lord Buddha and Lord Jesus Christ.

4. The *Vedas* are the oldest scriptures in the world. The essence of the *Vedas* is found in the *Bhagavad-gītā*, a literal record of Kṛṣṇa's words spoken five thousands years ago in India. The goal of Vedic knowledge—and of all religions—is to achieve love of God.

5. We can perfectly understand the knowledge of self-realization through the instructions of a genuine spiritual master—one who is free from selfish motives, who teaches the science of God explained in the *Bhagavad-gītā*, and whose mind is firmly fixed in meditation on Kṛṣṇa.

6. All that we eat should first be offered to Lord Kṛṣṇa with a prayer. In this way Kṛṣṇa accepts the offering and blesses it for our purification.

7. Rather than living in a self-centered way, we should act for the pleasure of Lord Kṛṣṇa. This is known as *bhakti-yoga*, the science of devotional service.

8. The most effective means for achieving God consciousness in this Age of Kali, or quarrel, is to chant the holy names of the Lord: Hare Kṛṣṇa, Hare Kṛṣṇa, Kṛṣṇa Kṛṣṇa, Hare Hare/ Hare Rāma, Hare Rāma, Rāma Rāma, Hare Hare.

Sanskrit Pronunciation Guide

The system of transliteration used in this book conforms to a system that scholars have accepted to indicate the pronunciation of each sound in the Sanskrit language.

The short vowel **a** is pronounced like the **u** in b**u**t, long **ā** like the **a** in f**a**r. Short **i** is pronounced as in p**i**n, long **ī** as in p**i**que, short **u** as in p**u**ll, and long **ū** as in r**u**le. The vowel **ṛ** is pronounced like the **ri** in **ri**m, **e** like the **ey** in th**ey**, **o** like the **o** in g**o**, **ai** like the **ai** in **ai**sle, and **au** like the **ow** in h**ow**. The *anusvāra* (**ṁ**) is pronounced like the **n** in the French word *bo***n**, and the *visarga* (**ḥ**) is pronounced as a final **h** sound. At the end of a couplet, **aḥ** is pronounced **aha** and **iḥ** is pronounced **ihi**.

The guttural consonants—**k, kh, g, gh,** and **ṅ**—are pronounced from the throat in much the same manner as in English. **K** is pronounced as in **k**ite, **kh** as in Ec**kh**art, **g** as in **g**ive, **gh** as in di**g h**ard, and **ṅ** as in si**ng.**

The palatal consonants—**c, ch, j, jh,** and **ñ**—are pronounced with the tongue touching the firm ridge behind the teeth. **C** is pronounced as in **ch**air, **ch** as in staun**ch-h**eart, **j** as in **j**oy, **jh** as in he**dgeh**og, and **ñ** as in ca**n**yon.

The cerebral consonants—**ṭ, ṭh, ḍ, ḍh,** and **ṇ**—are pronounced with the tip of the tongue turned up and drawn back against the dome of the palate. **Ṭ** is pronounced as in **t**ub, **ṭh** as in ligh**t-h**eart, **ḍ** as in **d**ove, **ḍh** as in re**d-h**ot, and **ṇ** as in **n**ut. The dental consonants—**t, th, d, dh,** and **n**—are pronounced in the same manner as the cerebrals, but with the forepart of the tongue against the teeth.

The labial consonants—**p, ph, b, bh,** and **m**—are pronounced with the lips. **P** is pronounced as in **p**ine, **ph** as in u**ph**ill, **b** as in **b**ird, **bh** as in ru**b-h**ard, and **m** as in **m**other.

The semivowels—**y, r, l,** and **v**—are pronounced as in **y**es, **r**un, **l**ight, and **v**ine respectively. The sibilants—**ś, ṣ,** and **s**—are pronounced, respectively, as in the German word **s***prechen* and the English words **sh**ine and **s**un. The letter **h** is pronounced as in **h**ome.

The International Society for Krishna Consciousness

Founder-Ācārya: His Divine Grace A.C. Bhaktivedanta Swami Prabhupāda

CENTERS AROUND THE WORLD

NORTH AMERICA

CANADA

Calgary, Alberta — 313 Fourth Street N.E., T2E 3S3/ Tel. (403) 265-3302

Edmonton, Alberta — 9353 35th Avenue, T6E 5R5/ Tel. (403) 439-9999

Montreal, Quebec — 1626 Pie IX Boulevard, H1V 2C5/ Tel. (514) 521-1301

Ottawa, Ontario — 212 Somerset St. E., K1N 6V4/ Tel. (613) 565-6544

Regina, Saskatchewan — 1279 Retallack St., S4T 2H8/ Tel. (306) 525-1640

Toronto, Ontario — 243 Avenue Rd., M5R 2J6/ Tel. (416) 922-5415

Vancouver, B.C. — 5462 S.E. Marine Dr., Burnaby V5J 3G8/ Tel. (604) 433-9728

Victoria, B.C. — 1350 Lang St., V8T 2S5/ Tel. (604) 920-0026

FARM COMMUNITY

Ashcroft, B.C. — Saranagati Dhama, Box 99, V0K 1A0

ADDITIONAL RESTAURANT

Vancouver — Hare Krishna Place, 46 Begbie St., New Westminster

U.S.A.

Atlanta, Georgia — 1287 South Ponce de Leon Ave. N.E., 30306/ Tel. (404) 378-9234

Baltimore, Maryland — 200 Bloomsbury Ave., Catonsville, 21228/ Tel. (410) 744-1624 or 4069

Boise, Idaho — 1615 Martha St., 83706/ Tel. (208) 344-4274

Boston, Massachusetts — 72 Commonwealth Ave., 02116/ Tel. (617) 247-8611

Chicago, Illinois — 1716 W. Lunt Ave., 60626/ Tel. (312) 973-0900

Columbus, Ohio — 379 W. Eighth Ave., 43201/ Tel. (614) 421-1661

Dallas, Texas — 5430 Gurley Ave., 75223/ Tel. (214) 827-6330

Denver, Colorado — 1400 Cherry St., 80220/ Tel. (303) 333-5461

Detroit, Michigan — 383 Lenox Ave., 48215/ Tel. (313) 824-6000

Gainesville, Florida — 214 N.W. 14th St., 32603/ Tel. (904) 336-4183

Gurabo, Puerto Rico — HC01-Box 8440, 00778-9763/ Tel. (809) 737-1658

Hartford, Connecticut — 1683 Main St., E. Hartford, 06108/ Tel. (860) 289-7252

Honolulu, Hawaii — 51 Coelho Way, 96817/ Tel. (808) 595-3947

Houston, Texas — 1320 W. 34th St., 77018/ Tel. (713) 686-4482

Laguna Beach, California — 285 Legion St., 92651/ Tel. (714) 494-7029

Long Island, New York — 197 S. Ocean Avenue, Freeport, 11520/ Tel. (516) 223-4909

Los Angeles, California — 3764 Watseka Ave., 90034/ Tel. (310) 836-2676

Miami, Florida — 3220 Virginia St., 33133 (mail: P.O. Box 337, Coconut Grove, FL 33233)/Tel. (305) 442-7218

New Orleans, Louisiana — 2936 Esplanade Ave., 70119/ Tel. (504) 486-3583

New York, New York — 305 Schermerhorn St., Brooklyn, 11217/ Tel. (718) 855-6714

New York, New York — 26 Second Avenue, 10003/ Tel. (212) 420-1130

Philadelphia, Pennsylvania — 41 West Allens Lane, 19119/ Tel. (215) 247-4600

Portland, Oregon — 5137 N.E. 42 Ave., 97218/ Tel. (503) 287-3252

St. Louis, Missouri — 3926 Lindell Blvd., 63108/ Tel. (314) 535-8085

San Diego, California — 1030 Grand Ave., Pacific Beach, 92109/ Tel. (619) 483-2500

Seattle, Washington — 1420 228th Ave. S.E., Issaquah, 98027/ Tel. (206) 391-3293

Tallahassee, Florida — 1323 Nylic St. (mail: P.O. Box 20224, 32304)/ Tel. (904) 681-9258

Towaco, New Jersey — P.O. Box 109, 07082/ Tel. (201) 299-0970

Tucson, Arizona — 711 E. Blacklidge Dr., 85719/ Tel. (520) 792-0630

Washington, D.C. — 3200 Ivy Way, Harwood, MD 20776/ Tel. (301) 261-4493

Washington, D.C. — 10310 Oaklyn Dr., Potomac, Maryland 20854/ Tel. (301) 299-2100

FARM COMMUNITIES

Alachua, Florida (New Raman Reti) — P.O. Box 819, 32615/ Tel. (904) 462-2017

Carriere, Mississippi (New Talavan) — 31492 Anner Road, 39426/ Tel. (601) 799-1354

Gurabo, Puerto Rico (New Govardhana Hill) — (contact ISKCON Gurabo)

Hillsborough, North Carolina (New Goloka) — 1032 Dimmocks Mill Rd., 27278/ Tel. (919) 732-6492

Mulberry, Tennessee (Murari-sevaka) — Rt. No. 1, Box 146-A, 37359/ Tel (615) 759-6888

Port Royal, Pennsylvania (Gita Nagari) — R.D. No. 1, Box 839, 17082/ Tel. (717) 527-4101

ADDITIONAL RESTAURANTS AND DINING

Boise, Idaho — Govinda's, 500 W. Main St., 83702/ Tel. (208) 338-9710

Eugene, Oregon — Govinda's Vegetarian Buffet, 270 W. 8th St., 97401/ Tel. (503) 686-3531

Fresno, California — Govinda's, 2373 E. Shaw, 93710/ Tel. (209) 225-1230

Gainesville, Florida — Radha's, 125 NW 23rd Ave., 32609/ Tel. (904) 376-9012

EUROPE

UNITED KINGDOM AND IRELAND

Belfast, Northern Ireland — 140 Upper Dunmurray Lane, BT17 OHE/ Tel. +44 (01232) 620530

Birmingham, England — 84 Stanmore Rd., Edgebaston, B16 9TB/ Tel. +44 (0121) 420-4999

Coventry, England — Sri Sri Radha Krishna Cultural Centre, Kingfield Rd., Radford (mail: 19 Gloucester St., CV1 3BZ)/ Tel. +44 (01203) 555420

Dublin, Ireland — 56 Dame St., Dublin 2/ Tel. +353 (01) 679-1306

Glasgow, Scotland — Karuna Bhavan, Bankhouse Rd., Lesmahagow, Lanarkshire ML11 0ES/Tel. +44 (01555) 894790

Leicester, England — 21 Thoresby St., North Evington, Leicester LE5 4GU/Tel. +44 (0116) 2762587 or 2367723

Liverpool, England — 114A Bold St., Liverpool L1 4HY/ Tel. +44 (0151) 708 9400
London, England (city) — 10 Soho St., London W1V 5DA/ Tel. +44 (0171) 4373662 (business hours), 4393606 (other times); Govinda's Restaurant: 4374928
London, England (country) — Bhaktivedanta Manor, Letchmore Heath, Watford, Hertfordshire WD2 8EP/ Tel. +44 (01923) 857244
London, England (south) — 42 Enmore Road, South Norwood, London SE25/ Tel. +44 (0181) 656-4296
Manchester, England — 20 Mayfield Rd., Whalley Range, Manchester M16 8FT/ Tel. +44 (0161) 2264416
Newcastle upon Tyne, England — 21 Leazes Park Rd., NE1 4PF/ Tel. +44 (0191) 2220150

FARM COMMUNITIES

County Wicklow, Ireland — Rathgorragh, Kiltegan/ Tel. +353 508-73305
Lisnaskea, North Ireland — Hare Krishna Island, BT92 9GN Lisnaskea, Co. Fremanagh/Tel. +44 (03657) 21512
London, England — (contact Bhaktivedanta Manor)

ADDITIONAL RESTAURANT

Manchester, England — Krishna's, 20 Cyril St., Manchester 14/ Tel. +44 (0161) 226 965
(Krishna conscious programs are held regularly in more than twenty other cities in the U.K. For information, contact Bhaktivedanta Books Ltd., Reader Services Dept., P.O. Box 324, Borehamwood, Herts WD6 1NB/ Tel. +44 [0181] 905-1244.)

GERMANY

Berlin — Johannisthaler Chaussee 78, 12259 Berlin (Britz)/ Tel. +49 (030) 613 2400
Boeblingen — Friedrich-List Strasse 58, 71032 Boeblingen/ Tel. +49 (07031) 22 33 98
Cologne — Taunusstr. 40, 51105 Köln/ Tel. +49 (0221) 830 3778
Flensburg— Hoerup 1, 24980 Neuhoerup/ Tel. +49 (04639) 73 36
Hamburg — Muehlenstr. 93, 25421 Pinneberg/ Tel. +49 (04101) 2 39 31
Hannover — Zeiss Strasse 21, 30519 Hannover/ Tel. +49 (0511) 83 74 31
Heidelberg — Kurfürsten-Anlage 5, D-69115 Heidelberg/ Tel. +49 (06221) 16 51 01
Munich — Tal 38, 80331 Munchen/ Tel +49 (089) 29 23 17
Nuremberg — Kopernikusplatz 12, 90459 Nürnberg/ Tel. +49 (0911) 45 32 86
Wiesbaden — Schiersteiner Strasse 6, 65187 Wiesbaden/ Tel. +49 (0611) 37 33 12

FARM COMMUNITY

Jandelsbrunn — Nava Jiyada Nrsimha Ksetra, Zielberg 20, 94118 Jandelsbrunn/ Tel +49 (08583) 316

ADDITIONAL RESTAURANT

Berlin — Higher Taste, Kurfuerstendamm 157/158, 10709 Berlin/ Tel. +49 (030) 892 99 17

ITALY

Asti — Roatto, Frazione Valle Reale 20/ Tel. +39 (0141) 938406
Bergamo — Villaggio Hare Krishna, Via Galileo Galilei 41, 24040 Chignolo D'isola (BG)/Tel. +39 (035) 4940706
Bologna — Via Ramo Barchetta 2, 40010 Bentivoglio (BO)/ Tel. +39 (051) 863924
Catania — Via San Nicolo al Borgo 28, 95128 Catania, Sicily/ Tel. +39 (095) 522-252
Naples — Via Vesuvio, N33, Ercolano LNA7/ Tel. +39 (081) 739-0398
Rome — Nepi, Sri Gaura Mandala, Via Mazzanese Km. 0,700 (dalla Cassia uscita Calcata), Pian del Pavone (Viterbo)/ Tel. +39 (0761) 527038
Vicenza — Via Roma 9, 36020 Albettone (Vicenza)/ Tel. +39 (0444) 790573 or 790566

FARM COMMUNITY

Florence (Villa Vrindavan) — Via Communale degli Scopeti 108, S. Andrea in Percussina, San Casciano, Val di Pesa (FI) 5002/ Tel. +39 (055) 820-054

ADDITIONAL RESTAURANT

Milan — Govinda's, Via Valpetrosa 3/5, 20123 Milano/ Tel. +39 (02) 862-417

POLAND

Augustow — ul Arnikowa 5, 16-300 Augustow/ Tel. & fax +48 (119) 46147
Bedzin — ul. Promyka 31, 42-500 Bedzin
Gdansk — ul. Cedrowa 5, Gdansk 80-125 (mail: MTSK 80-958 Gdansk 50 skr. poczt. 364)/ Tel. +48 (58) 329665
Krakow — ul. Podedworze 23a, 30-686 Krakow/ Tel. +48 (12) 588283
Lublin — ul Bursztynowa 12/52 (mail: Hare Kryszna, 20-001 Lublin 1, P.O. Box 196)/ Tel. +48 (81) 560685
Walbrzych — ul Schmidta 1/5, 58-300 Walbrzych/ Tel. +48 (74) 23185
Warsaw — Mysiadlo k. Warszawy, ul. Zakret 11, 05-500 Piaseczno (mail: MTSK 02-770 Warszawa 130, P.O. Box 257) / Tel. & fax +48 (22) 756-27-11
Wroclaw — ul. Bierutowska 23, 51-317 Wroclaw (mail: MTSK 50-900 Wroclaw, P.O. Box 858)/ Tel. & fax +48 (71) 250-981

FARM COMMUNITY

New Santipura — Czarnow 21, k. Kamiennej gory, woj. Jelenia gora/ Tel. +48 8745-1892

SWEDEN

Gothenburg — Hojdgatan 22, 431 36 Moelndal/ Tel. +46 (031) 879648
Grödinge — Korsnäs Gård, 14792 Grödinge/ Tel. +46 (8530) 29151
Karlstad — Vastra torgg. 16, 65224 Karlstad
Lund — Bredgatan 28 ipg, 222 21/ Tel. +46 (046) 120413
Malmö — Föreningsgatan 28, 21152 Malmö/ Tel. +46 (040) 6116497; restaurant: 6116496
Stockholm — Fridhemsgatan 22, 11240 Stockholm/ Tel. +46 (08) 6549 002
Uppsala — Nannaskolan sal F 3, Kungsgatan 22 (mail: Box 833, 751 08, Uppsala)/ Tel. +46 (018) 102924 or 509956

FARM COMMUNITY

Järna — Almviks Gård, 153 95 Järna/ Tel. +46 (8551) 52050; 52105

ADDITIONAL RESTAURANTS

Göthenburg — Govinda's, Storgatan 20,S-411 38 Göthenburg / Tel. +46 (031) 139698
Malmö — Higher Taste, Amiralsgatan 6, S-211 55 Malmö/ Tel. +46 (040) 970600
Umea — Govinda's, Pilg. 28, 90331 Umea/ Tel. +46 (090) 178875

SWITZERLAND

Basel — Hammerstrasse 11, 4058 Basel/ Tel. +41 (061) 693 26 38

Bern — Marktgasse 7, 3011 Bern/ Tel. +41 (031) 312 38 25
Lugano — Via ai Grotti, 6862 Rancate (TI)/ Tel. +41 (091) 646 66 16
Zürich — Bergstrasse 54, 8030 Zürich/ Tel. +41 (1) 262-33-88
Zürich — Preyergrasse 16, 8001 Zürich/ Tel. +41 (1) 251-88-59

OTHER COUNTRIES

Amsterdam, The Netherlands — Van Hilligaertstraat 17, 1072 JX, Amsterdam/ Tel. +31 (020) 6751404
Antwerp, Belgium — Amerikalei 184, 2000 Antwerpen/ Tel. +32 (03) 237-0037
Barcelona, Spain — c/de L'Oblit 67, 08026 Barcelona/ Tel. +34 (93) 347-9933
Belgrade, Serbia — VVZ-Veda, Custendilska 17, 11000 Beograd/ Tel. +381 (11) 781-695
Budapest, Hungary — Hare Krishna Temple, Mariaremetei ut. 77, Budapest 1028 II/Tel. +36 (01) 1768774
Copenhagen, Denmark — Baunevej 23, 3400 Hillerød/ Tel. +45 42286446
Debrecen, Hungary — L. Hegyi Mihalyne, U62, Debrecen 4030/ Tel. +36 (052) 342-496
Helsinki, Finland — Ruoholahdenkatu 24 D (III krs) 00180, Helsinki/ Tel. +358 (0) 6949879
Iasi, Romania — Stradela Moara De Vint 72, 6600 Iasi
Kaunas, Lithuania — Savanoryu 37, Kaunas/ Tel. +370 (07) 222574
Ljubljana, Slovenia — Zibertova 27, 61000 Ljubljana/ Tel. +386 (061) 131-23-19
Madrid, Spain — Espíritu Santo 19, 28004 Madrid/ Tel. +34 (91) 521-3096
Málaga, Spain — Ctra. Alora, 3 int., 29140 Churriana/ Tel. +34 (952) 621038
Oslo, Norway — Jonsrudvej 1G, 0274 Oslo/ Tel. +47 (022) 552243
Paris, France — 31 Rue Jean Vacquier, 93160 Noisy le Grand/ Tel. +33 (01) 43043263
Plovdiv, Bulgaria — ul. Prosveta 56, Kv. Proslav, Plovdiv 4015/ Tel. +359 (032) 446962
Porto, Portugal — Rua S. Miguel, 19 C.P. 4000 (mail: Apartado 4108, 4002 Porto Codex)/ Tel. +351 (02) 2005469
Prague, Czech Republic — Jilova 290, Prague 5-Zlicin 155 00/ Tel. +42 (02) 3021282 or 3021608
Pula, Croatia — Vinkuran centar 58, 52000 Pula (mail: P.O. Box 16)/ Tel. & fax +385 (052) 573581
Rijeka, Croatia — Svetog Jurja 32, 51000 Rijeka (mail: P.O. Box 61)/ Tel. & fax +385 (051) 263404
Riga, Latvia — 56 Krishyana Barona, LV 1011/ Tel. +371 (02) 272490
Rotterdam, The Netherlands — Braamberg 45, 2905 BK Capelle a/d Yssel./ Tel. +31 (010) 4580873
Santa Cruz de Tenerife, Spain — C/ Castillo, 44, 4°, Santa Cruz 38003,Tenerife/ Tel. +34 (922) 241035
Sarajevo, Bosnia-Herzegovina — Saburina 11, 71000 Sarajevo/ Tel. +381 (071) 531-154
Septon-Durbuy, Belgium — Chateau de Petite Somme, 6940 Septon-Durbuy/ Tel. +32 (086) 322926
Skopje, Macedonia — Vvz. "ISKCON," Roze Luksemburg 13, 91000 Skopje/ Tel. +389 (091) 201451
Sofia, Bulgaria — Villa 3, Vilna Zona-Iztok, Simeonovo, Sofia 1434/ Tel. +359 (02) 6352608
Split, Croatia — Cesta Mutogras 26, 21312 Podstrana, Split (mail: P.O. Box 290, 21001 Split)/ Tel. +385 (021) 651137
Tallinn, Estonia — ul Linnamae Tee 11-97/ Tel. +372 (0142) 59756
Timisoara, Romania — ISKCON, Porumbescu 92, 1900 Timisoara/ Tel. +40 (961) 54776
Vienna, Austria — ISKCON, Rosenackerstrasse 26, 1170 Vienna/ Tel. +43 (01) 455830
Vilnius, Lithuania — Raugyklos G. 23-1, 2024 Vilnius/ Tel. +370 (0122) 66-12-18
Zagreb, Croatia — Bizek 5,10000 Zagreb (mail: P.O. Box 68, 10001 Zagreb)/ Tel. & fax +385 (01) 190548

FARM COMMUNITIES

Czech Republic — Krsnuv Dvur c. 1, 257 28 Chotysany
France (Bhaktivedanta Village) — Chateau Bellevue, F-39700 Chatenois/ Tel. +33 (084) 728235
France (La Nouvelle Mayapura) — Domaine d'Oublaisse, 36360, Lucay le Mâle/ Tel. +33 (054) 402481
Spain (New Vraja Mandala) — (Santa Clara) Brihuega, Guadalajara/ Tel. +34 (911) 280018

ADDITIONAL RESTAURANTS

Barcelona, Spain — Restaurante Govinda, Plaza de la Villa de Madrid 4-5, 08002 Barcelona
Copenhagen, Denmark — Govinda's, Noerre Farimagsgade 82/ Tel. +45 33337444
Oslo, Norway — Krishna's Cuisine, Kirkeveien 59B, 0364 Oslo/ Tel. +47 22606250
Prague, Czech Republic — Govinda's, Soukenicka 27, 110 00 Prague-1/ Tel. +42 (02) 2481-6631, 2481-6016
Prague, Czech Republic — Govinda's, Na hrazi 5, 180 00 Prague 8-Liben/ Tel. +42 (02) 683-7226
Vienna, Austria — Govinda, Lindengasse 2A, 1070 Vienna/ Tel. +43 (01) 5222817

COMMONWEALTH OF INDEPENDENT STATES

RUSSIA

Moscow — Khoroshevskoye shosse d.8, korp.3, 125 284, Moscow/ Tel. +7 (095) 255-67-11
Moscow — Nekrasovsky pos., Dmitrovsky reg., 141760 Moscow/ Tel. +7 (095) 979-8268
Nijni Novgorod — ul. Ivana Mochalova, 7-69, 603904 Nijni Novgorod/ Tel. +7 (8312) 252592
Novosibirsk — ul. Leningradskaya 111-20, Novosibirsk
Perm (Ural Region) — Pr. Mira, 113-142, 614065 Perm/ Tel. +7 (3442) 335740
St. Petersburg — 17, Bumazhnaya st., 198020 St. Petersburg/ Tel. +7 (0812) 186-7259
Ulyanovsk — ul Glinki, 10 /Tel. +7 (0842) 221-42-89
Vladivostok — ul. Ridneva 5-1, 690087 Vladivostok/ Tel. +7 (4232) 268943

UKRAINE

Dnepropetrovsk — ul. Ispolkomovskaya, 56A, 320029 Dnepropetrovsk/ Tel. +380 (0562) 445029
Donetsk — ul. Tubensa, 22, 339018 Makeyevka/ Tel. +380 (0622) 949104
Kharkov — ul. Verhnyogievskaya, 43, 310015 Kharkov/Tel. +380 (0572) 202167 or 726968
Kiev — ul. Menjinskogo, 21-B., 252054 Kiev/Tel. +380 (044) 2444944
Nikolayev — Sudostroitelny pereulok, 5/8, Nikolayev 327052/ Tel. +380 (0512) 351734
Simferopol — ul. Kievskaya 149/15, 333000 Simferopol/ Tel. +380 (0652) 225116
Vinnitza — ul. Chkalov St., 5, Vinnitza 26800/ Tel. +380 (0432) 323152

OTHER COUNTRIES

Alma Ata, Kazakstan — Per Kommunarov, 5, 480022 Alma Ata/ Tel. +7 (3272) 353830
Baku, Azerbaijan — Pos. 8-i km, per. Sardobi 2, Baku 370060/ Tel. +7 (8922) 212376

Bishkek, Kyrgizstan — Per. Omski, 5, 720000 Bishkek/ Tel. +7 (3312) 472683
Dushanbe, Tadjikistan — ul Anzob, 38, 724001 Dushanbe/ Tel. +7 (3772) 271830
Kishinev, Moldova — ul. Popovich 13, Kishinev/ Tel. +7 (0422) 558099
Minsk, Belarus — ul. Pavlova 11, 220 053 Minsk/ Tel. +7 (0172) 37-4751
Sukhumi, Georgia — Pr. Mira 274, Sukhumi
Tbilisi, Georgia — ul. Kacharava, 16, 380044 Tbilisi/ Tel. +7 (8832) 623326
Yerevan, Armenia — ul. Krupskoy 18, 375019 Yerevan/ Tel. +7 (8852) 275106

AUSTRALASIA

AUSTRALIA

Canberra — 15 Parkhill St., Pearce ACT 2607 (mail: GPO Box 1411, Canberra 2601)/ Tel. +61 (06) 290-1869
Melbourne — 197 Danks St., Albert Park, Victoria 3206 (mail: P.O. Box 125)/ Tel. +61 (03) 969 95122
Perth — 356 Murray St., Perth (mail: P.O. Box 102, Bayswater, W. A. 6053)/ Tel. +61 (09) 481-1114 or 370-1552 (evenings)
Sydney — 180 Falcon St., North Sydney, N.S.W. 2060 (mail: P. O. Box 459, Cammeray, N.S.W.2062)/ Tel. +61 (02) 9959-4558
Sydney — 3296 King St., Newtown 2042/ Tel. +61 (02) 550-6524

FARM COMMUNITIES

Bambra (New Nandagram) — Oak Hill, Dean's Marsh Rd., Bambra, VIC 3241/ Tel. +61 (052) 88-7383
Millfield, N.S.W. — New Gokula Farm, Lewis Lane (off Mt.View Rd. Millfield near Cessnock), N.S.W. (mail: P.O. Box 399, Cessnock 2325, N.S.W.)/ Tel. +61 (049) 98-1800
Murwillumbah (New Govardhana) — Tyalgum Rd., Eungella, via Murwillumbah N. S. W. 2484 (mail: P.O. Box 687)/ Tel. +61 (066) 72-6579

ADDITIONAL RESTAURANTS

Adelaide — Food for Life, 79 Hindley St./ Tel. +61 (08) 2315258
Brisbane — Govinda's, 1st floor, 99 Elizabeth Street/ Tel. +61 (07) 210-0255
Brisbane — Hare Krishna Food for Life, 190 Brunswick St. Fortitude Valley/ Tel. +61 (070) 854-1016
Melbourne — Crossways, Floor 1, 123 Swanston St., Melbourne, Victoria 3000/ Tel. +61 (03) 9650-2939
Melbourne — Gopal's, 139 Swanston St., Melbourne, Victoria 3000/ Tel. +61 (03) 9650-1578
Perth — Hare Krishna Food for Life, 200 William St., Northbridge, WA 6003/ Tel. +61 (09) 227-1684

NEW ZEALAND, FIJI, AND PAPUA NEW GUINEA

Christchurch, New Zealand — 83 Bealey Ave. (mail: P.O. Box 25-190 Christchurch)/ Tel. +64 (03) 3665-174
Labasa, Fiji — Delailabasa (mail: P.O. Box 133)/ Tel. +679 812912
Lautoka, Fiji — 5 Tavewa Ave. (mail: P.O. Box 125)/ Tel. +679 664112
Port Moresby, Papua New Guinea — Section 23, Lot 46, Gordonia St., Hohola (mail: P. O. Box 571, POM NCD)/ Tel. +675 259213
Rakiraki, Fiji — Rewasa, Rakiraki (mail: P.O. Box 204)/ Tel. +679 694243
Suva, Fiji — Nasinu 7½ miles (mail: P.O. Box 7315)/ Tel. +679 393599
Wellington, New Zealand — 60 Wade St., Wadestown, Wellington (mail: P.O. Box 2753, Wellington)/ Tel. +64 (04) 4720510

FARM COMMUNITY

Auckland, New Zealand (New Varshan) — Hwy. 18, Riverhead, next to Huapai Golf Course (mail: R.D. 2, Kumeu, Auckland)/ Tel. +64 (09) 4128075

RESTAURANTS

Auckland, New Zealand — Gopal's, Civic House (1st floor), 291 Queen St./ Tel. +64 (09) 3034885
Christchurch, New Zealand — Gopal's, 143 Worcester St./ Tel. +64 (03) 3667-035
Labasa, Fiji — Hare Krishna Restaurant, Naseakula Road/ Tel. +679 811364
Lautoka, Fiji — Gopal's, Corner of Yasawa St. and Naviti St./ Tel. +679 662990
Suva, Fiji — Gopal's, 18 Pratt St./ Tel. +679 314154

AFRICA

NIGERIA

Abeokuta — Ibadan Rd., Obanatoka (mail: P.O. Box 5177)
Benin City — 108 Lagos Rd., Uselu/ Tel. +234 (052) 247900
Enugu — 8 Church Close, off College Rd., Housing Estate, Abakpa-Nike
Ibadan — 1 Ayo Akintoba St., Agbowo, University of Ibadan
Jos — 5A Liberty Dam Close, P.O. Box 6557, Jos
Kaduna — 8B Dabo Rd., Kaduna South, P.O. Box 1121, Kaduna
Lagos — 25 Jaiyeola Ajata St., Ajao Estate, off International Airport Express Rd., Lagos (mail: P.O. Box 8793)/ Tel. & Fax +234 (01) 876169
Port Harcourt — Second Tarred Road, Ogwaja Waterside (mail: P.O. Box 4429, Trans Amadi)
Warri — Okwodiete Village, Kilo 8, Effurun/Orerokpe Rd. (mail: P.O. Box 1922, Warri)

SOUTH AFRICA

Cape Town — 17 St. Andrews Rd., Rondebosch 7700/ Tel. +27 (021) 689-1529
Durban — Chatsworth Centre, Chatsworth 4030 (mail: P.O. Box 56003)/ Tel. +27 (31) 433-328
Johannesburg — 14 Goldreich St., Hillbrow 2001 (mail: P.O. Box 10667, Johannesburg 2000)/ Tel. +27 (011) 484-3273
Port Elizabeth — 18 Strand Fontein Rd., 6001 Port Elizabeth/ Tel. & Fax +27 (41) 53 43 30

OTHER COUNTRIES

Gaborone, Botswana — P.O. Box 201003/ Tel. +267 307 768
Kampala, Uganda — Bombo Rd., near Makerere University (mail: P.O. Box 1647, Kampala)
Kisumu, Kenya — P.O. Box 547/ Tel. +254 (035) 42546
Marondera, Zimbabwe — 6 Pine Street (mail: P.O. Box 339)/ Tel. +263 (028) 8877801
Mombasa, Kenya — Hare Krishna House, Sauti Ya Kenya and Kisumu Rds. (mail: P.O. Box 82224, Mombasa)/ Tel. +254 (011) 312248
Nairobi, Kenya — Muhuroni Close, off West Nagara Rd. (mail: P.O. Box 28946, Nairobi)/ Tel. +254 (02) 744365
Phoenix, Mauritius — Hare Krishna Land, Pont Fer, Phoenix (mail: P. O. Box 108, Quartre Bornes, Mauritius)/ Tel. +230 696-5804
Rose Hill, Mauritius — 13 Gordon St./ Tel. +230 454-5275

FARM COMMUNITY

Mauritius (ISKCON Vedic Farm) — Hare Krishna Rd., Vrindaban, Bon Acceuil/ Tel. +230 418-3955

ASIA

INDIA

Agartala, Tripura — Assam-Agartala Rd., Banamalipur, 799001

Ahmedabad, Gujarat — Sattelite Rd., Gandhinagar Highway Crossing, Ahmedabad 380054/ Tel. (079) 6749827, 6749945

Allahabad, U. P. — 161, Kashi Nagar, Baluaghat, Allahabad 211003/ Tel. 653318

Bamanbore, Gujarat — N.H. 8A, Surendra-nagar District

Bangalore, Karnataka — Hare Krishna Hill, 1 'R' Block, Chord Road, Rajaji Nagar 560010/ Tel. (080) 332 1956

Baroda, Gujarat — Hare Krishna Land, Gotri Rd., 390021/ Tel. (0265) 326299 or 331012

Belgaum, Karnataka — Shukravar Peth, Tilak Wadi, 590006

Bhubaneswar, Orissa — National Highway No. 5, Nayapali, 751001/ Tel. (0674) 413517 or 413475

Bombay — (see Mumbai)

Calcutta, W. Bengal — 3C Albert Rd., 700017/ Tel. (033) 2473757 or 2476075

Chandigarh — Hare Krishna Land, Dakshin Marg, Sector 36-B, 160036/ Tel. (0172) 601590 and 603232

Coimbatore, Tamil Nadu — 387, VGR Puram, Dr. Alagesan Rd., 641011/ Tel. (0422) 445978 or 442749

Gangapur, Gujarat — Bhaktivedanta Rajavidyalaya, Krishnalok, Surat-Bardoli Rd. Gangapur, P.O. Gangadhara, Dist. Surat, 394310/Tel. (02,61) 667075

Gauhati, Assam — Ulubari Charali, Gauhati 781001/ Tel. (0361) 31208

Guntur, A.P. — Opp. Sivalayam, Peda Kakani 522509

Hanumkonda, A.P. — Neeladri Rd., Kapuwada, 506011/ Tel. 08712-77399

Haridwar, U.P. — ISKCON, P.O. Box 4, Haridwar, U.P. 249401/ Tel. (0133) 422655

Hyderabad, A.P. — Hare Krishna Land, Nampally Station Rd., 500001/ Tel. (040) 592018 or 552924

Imphal, Manipur — Hare Krishna Land, Airport Road, 795001/ Tel. (0385) 221587

Jaipur, Rajasthan — P.O. Box 270, Jaipur 302001/ Tel. (0141) 364022

Katra, Jammu, and Kashmir — Srila Prabhupada Ashram, Srila Prabhupada Marg, Kalka Mata Mandir, Katra (Vashnov Mata) 182101/ Tel. (01991) 3047

Kurukshetra, Haryana — 369 Gudri Muhalla, Main Bazaar, 132118/ Tel. (1744) 32806 or 33529

Lucknow, Uttar Pradesh — 1 Ashak Nagar, Guru Govind Singh Marg, 226018

Madras, Tamil Nadu — 59, Burkit Rd., T. Nagar, 600017/ Tel. 443266

Mayapur, W. Bengal — Shree Mayapur Chandrodaya Mandir, Shree Mayapur Dham, Dist. Nadia (mail: P.O. Box 10279, Ballyganj, Calcutta 700019)/ Tel. (03472) 45239 or 45240 or 45233

Moirang, Manipur — Nongban Ingkhon, Tidim Rd./ Tel. 795133

Mumbai, Maharashtra (Bombay) — Hare Krishna Land, Juhu 400 049/ Tel. (022) 6206860

Mumbai, Maharashtra — 7 K. M. Munshi Marg, Chowpatty, 400007/ Tel. (022) 3634078

Mumbai, Maharashtra — Shivaji Chowk, Station Rd., Bhayandar (West), Thane 401101/ Tel. (022) 8191920

Nagpur, Maharashtra — 70 Hill Road, Ramnagar, 440010/ Tel. (0712) 529932

New Delhi — Sant Nagar Main Road (Garhi), behind Nehru Place Complex (mail: P. O. Box 7061), 110065/ Tel. (011) 6419701 or 6412058

New Delhi — 14/63, Punjabi Bagh, 110026/ Tel. (011) 5410782

Pandharpur, Maharashtra — Hare Krsna Ashram (across Chandrabhaga River), Dist. Sholapur, 413304/ Tel. (0218) 623473

Patna, Bihar — Rajendra Nagar Road No. 12, 800016/ Tel. (0612) 50765

Pune, Maharashtra — 4 Tarapoor Rd., Camp, 411001/ Tel. (0212) 667259

Puri, Orissa — Sipasurubuli Puri, Dist. Puri/ (06752) 24592, 24594

Puri, Orissa — Bhakti Kuthi, Swargadwar, Puri/ Tel. (06752) 23740

Secunderabad, A.P. — 27 St. John's Road, 500026/ Tel. (040) 805232

Silchar, Assam — Ambikapatti, Silchar, Cachar Dist., 788004

Siliguri, W. Bengal — Gitalpara, 734401/ Tel. (0353) 26619

Surat, Gujarat — Rander Rd., Jahangirpura, 395005/ Tel. (0261) 685516 or 685891

Sri Rangam, Tamal Nadu — 6A E.V.S. Rd., Sri Rangam, Tiruchirapalli 6/ Tel. 433945

Tirupati, A. P. — K.T. Road, Vinayaka Nagar, 517507/ Tel. (08574) 20114

Trivandrum, Kerala — T.C. 224/1485, WC Hospital Rd., Thycaud, 695014/ Tel. (0471) 68197

Udhampur, Jammu and Kashmir — Srila Prabhupada Ashram, Prabhupada Marg, Prabhupada Nagar, Udhampur 182101/ Tel. (01992) 70298

Vallabh Vidyanagar, Gujarat — ISKCON Hare Krishna Land, 338120/ Tel. (02692) 30796

Vrindavana, U. P. — Krishna-Balaram Mandir, Bhaktivedanta Swami Marg, Raman Reti, Mathura Dist., 281124/ Tel. (0565) 442-478 or 442-355

FARM COMMUNITIES

Ahmedabad District, Gujarat — Hare Krishna Farm, Katwada (contact ISKCON Ahmedabad)

Assam — Karnamadhu, Dist. Karimganj

Chamorshi, Maharashtra — 78 Krishnanagar Dham, Dis. Gadhachiroli, 442603

OTHER COUNTRIES

Cagayan de Oro, Philippines — 30 Dahlia St., Ilaya Carmen, 900 (c/o Sepulveda's Compound)

Chittagong, Bangladesh — Caitanya Cultural Society, Sri Pundarik Dham, Mekhala, Hathzari (mail: GPO Box 877, Chittagong)/ Tel. +88 (031) 225822

Colombo, Sri Lanka — 188 New Chetty St., Colombo 13/ Tel. +94 (01) 433325

Dhaka, Bangladesh — 5 Chandra Mohon Basak St., Banagram, Dhaka 1203/ Tel. +880 (02) 236249

Hong Kong — 27 Chatam Road South, 6/F, Kowloon/ Tel. +852 7396818

Iloilo City, Philippines — 13-1-1 Tereos St., La Paz, Iloilo City, Iloilo/ Tel. +63 (033) 73391

Jakarta, Indonesia — P.O. Box 2694, Jakarta Pusat 10001/ Tel. +62 (021) 4899646

Jessore, Bangladesh — Nitai Gaur Mandir, Kathakhali Bazaar, P. O. Panjia, Dist. Jessore

Jessore, Bangladesh — Rupa-Sanatana Smriti Tirtha, Ramsara, P. O. Magura Hat, Dist. Jessore

Kathmandu, Nepal — Budhanilkantha, Kathmandu (mail: P. O. Box 3520)/ Tel. +977 (01) 290743

Kuala Lumpur, Malaysia — Lot 9901, Jalan Awan Jawa, Taman Yarl, off 5½ Mile, Jalan Kelang Lama, Petaling/ Tel. +60 (03) 780-7355, -7360, or -7369
Manila, Philippines — Penthouse Liwag Bldg., 3307 Mantanzas St., Makati, Metro Manila/ Tel. +63 (02) 8337883 loc. 10
Taipei, Taiwan — (mail: c/o ISKCON Hong Kong)
Tel Aviv, Israel — 16 King George St. (mail: P. O. Box 48163, Tel Aviv 61480)/ Tel. +972 (03) 5285475 or 6299011
Tokyo, Japan — 1-29-2-202 Izumi, Suginami-ku, Tokyo 168/ Tel. +81 (03) 3327-1541
Yogyakarta, Indonesia — P.O. Box 25, Babarsari YK, DIY

FARM COMMUNITIES

Indonesia — Govinda Kunja (contact ISKCON Jakarta)
Malaysia — Jalan Sungai Manik, 36000 Teluk Intan, Perak
Philippines (Hare Krishna Paradise) — 231 Pagsabungan Rd., Basak, Mandaue City/ Tel. +63 (032) 83254

ADDITIONAL RESTAURANTS

Cebu, Philippines — Govinda's, 26 Sanchiangko St.
Kuala Lumpur, Malaysia — Govinda's, 16-1 Jalan Bunus Enam, Masjid India/ Tel. +60 (03) 7807355 or 7807360 or 7807369

LATIN AMERICA

BRAZIL

Belém, PA — Almirante Barroso, Travessa Santa Matilde, 64, Souza/ Tel. +55 (091) 243-0558
Belo Horizonte, MG — Rua Aristoteles Caldeira, 334, Prado/ Tel. +55 (031) 332-8460
Brasilia, DF — CLN 310, Bloco B, Loja 45, Terreo/ Tel. +55 (061) 272-3111
Campos, RJ — Rua Barao de Miracema, 186, Centro
Caruaru, PE — Rua Major Sinval, 180, 1° Andar
Curitiba, PR — Al. Cabral, 670, Centro/ Tel. +55 (041) 277-3176
Florianopolis, SC — Rua Laurindo Januario Silveira, 3250, Canto da Lagoa
Fortaleza, CE — Rua Jose Lourenço, 2114, Aldeota/ Tel. +55 (085) 264-1273
Goiania, GO — Rua 24A, 20 (esq. Av. Parananba)/ Tel. +55 (062) 224-9820
Guarulhos, SP — Rua Orixas, 1, Jardim Afonso/ Tel. +55 (011) 209-6669
Manaus, AM — Av. 7 de Setembro, 1599, Centro/ Tel. +55 (092) 232-0202
Petropolis, RJ — Rua do Imperador, 349, Sobrado
Porto Alegre, RS — Av. Basian, 396, Menino Deus/ Tel. +55 (051) 233-1474
Recife, PE — Rua Democlitos de Souza Filho, 235, Madalena
Ribeirao Preto, SP — Rua dos Aliados, 155, Campos Eliseos/ Tel. +55 (016) 628-1533
Rio de Janeiro, RJ — Rua Barao da Torre, 199, apt. 102, Ipanema/ Tel. +55 (021) 267-0052
Salvador, BA — Rua Alvaro Adorno, 17, Brotas/ Tel. +55 (071) 382-1064
Santos, SP — Rua Nabuco de Araujo, 151, Embare/ Tel. +55 (0132) 38-4655
São Carlos, SP — Rua Emilio Ribas, 195
São Paulo, SP — Av. Angelica, 2583/Tel. +55 (011) 259-7352
São Paulo, SP — Rua Otavio Tarquino de Souza, 299, Congonhas/ Tel. +55 (011) 536-4010

FARM COMMUNITIES

Autazes, AM — Nova Jarikandha/ Tel. +55 (092) 232-0202
Caruaru, PE — Nova Vrajadhama, Distrito de Murici, CP 283, CEP 55000-000
Curitiba, PR — Nova Goloka, Planta Carla, Pinhais
Parati, RJ — Goura Vrindavan, Bairro de Grauna, CP 062, CEP 23970-000
Pindamonhangaba, SP — Nova Gokula, Bairro Ribeiro Grande, CP 108, CEP 12400-000/ Tel. +55 (012) 982-9036
Teresopolis, RJ — Vrajabhumi, Canoas, CP 92687, CEP 25951-970

MEXICO

Guadalajara — Pedro Moreno No. 1791, Sector Juarez/ Tel. +52 (38) 160775
Mexico City — Gob. Tiburcio Montiel No. 45, 11850 Mexico, D.F./ Tel. +52 (5) 271-22-23
Saltillo — Blvd. Saltillo No. 520, Col. Buenos Aires

FARM COMMUNITY

Guadalajara — Contact ISKCON Guadalajara

ADDITIONAL RESTAURANTS

Orizaba — Restaurante Radhe, Sur 5 No. 50, Orizaba, Ver./ Tel. +52 (272) 5-75-25

PERU

Lima — Pasaje Solea 101 Santa Maria-Chosica/ Tel. +51 (014) 910891
Lima — Schell 634 Miraflores
Lima — Av. Garcilazo de la Vega 1670-1680/ Tel. +51 (014) 259523

FARM COMMUNITY

Correo De Bella Vista — DPTO De San Martin

ADDITIONAL RESTAURANT

Cuzco — Espaderos 128

OTHER COUNTRIES

Asunción, Paraguay — Centro Bhaktivedanta, Mariano R. Alonso 925, Asunción/ Tel. +595 (021) 480-266
Bogotá, Colombia — Calle 72, nro.20-60, Bogota (mail: Apartado Aereo 58680, Zona 2, Chapinero)/ Tel. & Fax +57 (01) 2554529, 2482234
Buenos Aires, Argentina — Centro Bhaktivedanta, Andonaegui 2054 (1431)/ Tel. +54 (01) 521- 5567, 523-4232
Cali, Colombia — Avenida 2 EN, #24N-39/ Tel. +57 (023) 68-88-53
Caracas, Venezuela — Avenida Berlin, Quinta Tia Lola, La California Norte/ Tel. +58 (02) 225463
Chinandega, Nicaragua — Edificio Hare Krsna No. 108, Del Banco Nacional 10 mts. abajo/ Tel. +505 (341) 2359
Cochabamba, Bolivia — Av. Heroinas E-0435 Apt. 3 (mail: P. O. Box 2070)/ Tel. & Fax +591 (042) 54346
Essequibo Coast, Guyana — New Navadvipa Dham, Mainstay, Essequibo Coast
Georgetown, Guyana — 24 Uitvlugt Front, West Coast Demerara
Guatemala, Guatemala — Apartado Postal 1534
Guayaquil, Ecuador — 6 de Marzo 226 or V. M. Rendon/ Tel. +593 (04) 308412 y 309420
Managua, Nicaragua — Residencial Bolonia, De Galeria los Pipitos 75 mts. norte (mail: P.O. Box 772)/ Tel. +505 242759

Mar del Plata, Argentina — Dorrego 4019 (7600) Mar del Plata/ Tel. +54 (023) 745688
Montevideo, Uruguay — Centro de Bhakti-Yoga, Mariano Moreno 2660, Montevideo/ Tel. +598 (02) 477919
Panama, Republic of Panama — Via las Cumbres, entrada Villa Zaita, frente a INPSA No.1 (mail: P.O. Box 6-29-54, Panama)
Pereira, Colombia — Carrera 5a, #19-36
Quito, Ecuador — Inglaterra y Amazonas
Rosario, Argentina — Centro de Bhakti-Yoga, Paraguay 556, (2000) Rosario/ Tel. +54 (041) 252630, 264243
San José, Costa Rica — Centro Cultural Govinda, Av. 7, Calles 1 y 3, 235 mtrs. norte del Banco Anglo, San Pedro (mail: Apdo. 166,1002)/ Tel. +5206 23-52 38
San Salvador, El Salvador — Avenida Universitaria 1132, Media Quadra al sur de la Embajada Americana (mail: P.O. Box 1506)/ Tel. +503 25-96-17
Santiago, Chile — Carrera 330/ Tel. +56 (02) 698-8044
Santo Domingo, Dominican Republic — Calle Cayetano Rodriquez No. 254/ Tel. (809) 686-5665
Trinidad and Tobago, West Indies — Orion Drive, Debe/ Tel. +1 (809) 647-3165
Trinidad and Tobago, West Indies — Prabhupada Ave. Longdenville, Chaguanas

FARM COMMUNITIES

Argentina (Bhaktilata Puri) — Casilla de Correo No 77, 1727 Marcos Paz, Pcia. Bs. As., Republica Argentina
Bolivia — Contact ISKCON Cochabamba
Colombia (Nueva Mathura) — Cruzero del Guali, Municipio de Caloto, Valle del Cauca/ Tel. 612688 en Cali
Costa Rica — Nueva Goloka Vrindavana, Carretera a Paraiso, de la entrada del Jardin Lancaster (por Calle Concava), 200 metros al sur (mano derecha) Cartago (mail: Apdo. 166, 1002)/ Tel. +506 551-6752
Ecuador (Nueva Mayapur) — Ayampe (near Guayaquil)
Ecuador (Giridharidesha) — Chordeleg (near Cuenca), Cassiga Postal 01.05.1811, Cuenca/ Tel. +593 (7) 255735
El Salvador — Carretera a Santa Ana, Km. 34, Canton Los Indios, Zapotitan, Dpto. de La Libertad
Guyana — Seawell Village, Corentyne, East Berbice

ADDITIONAL RESTAURANTS

Buenos Aires, Argentina — Gusto Superior, Blanco Encalada 2722, 1428 Buenos Aires Cap. Fed./ Tel. +54 (01) 788 3023
Cochabamba, Bolivia — Gopal Restaurant, calle España N-0250 (Galeria Olimpia) (mail: P. O. Box 2070, Cochabamba)/ Tel. +591 (042) 26626
Guatemala, Guatemala — Callejor Santandes a una cuadra abajo de Guatel, Panajachel Solola
San Salvador, El Salvador — 25 Avenida Norte 1132
Santa Cruz, Bolivia — Snack Govinda, Av. Argomosa (1ero anillo), esq. Bolivar/ Tel. +591 (03) 345189

BHAGAVAD-GĪTĀ AS IT IS

The world's most popular edition of a timeless classic.

Throughout the ages, the world's greatest minds have turned to the *Bhagavad-gītā* for answers to life's perennial questions. Renowned as the jewel of India's spiritual wisdom, the *Gītā* summarizes the profound Vedic knowledge concerning man's essential nature, his environment, and ultimately his relationship with God. With more than fifty million copies sold in twenty languages, *Bhagavad-gītā As It Is,* by His Divine Grace A.C. Bhaktivedanta Swami Prabhupāda, is the most widely read edition of the *Gītā* in the world. It includes the original Sanskrit text, phonetic transliterations, word-for-word meanings, translation, elaborate commentary, and many full-color illustrations. (Pocket version: translation and commentary only.)

Pocket	Vinyl	Hard	Deluxe
$4.50	$8.50	$9.95	$19.95
BGS	BGV	BGH	BGD

ORDER TOLL FREE 1-800-927-4152

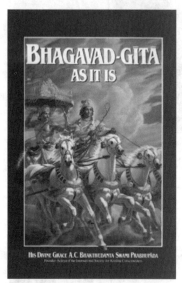

GREAT
VEGETARIAN DISHES

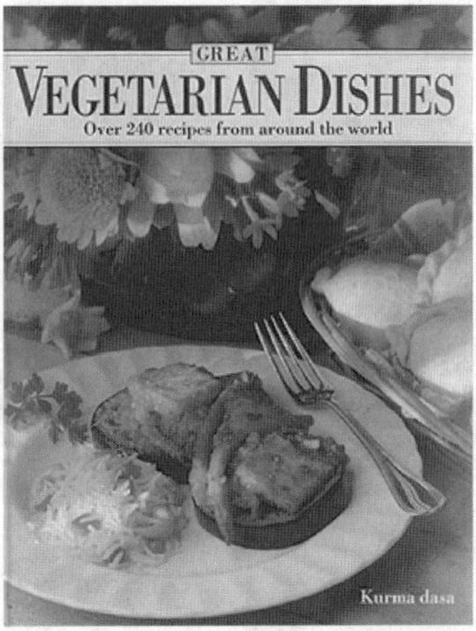

Featuring over 100 stunning full-color photos, this new book is for spiritually aware people who want the exquisite taste of Hare Krishna cooking without a lot of time in the kitchen. The 240 international recipes were tested and refined by world-famous Hare Krishna chef Kurma dasa.

240 recipes, 192 pages, coffee-table-size hardback

US: $19.95 #GVD

THE HARE KRISHNA BOOK OF
VEGETARIAN COOKING

A colorfully illustrated, practical cookbook that not only helps you prepare authentic Indian dishes at home but also teaches you about the ancient tradition behind India's world-famous vegetarian cuisine.

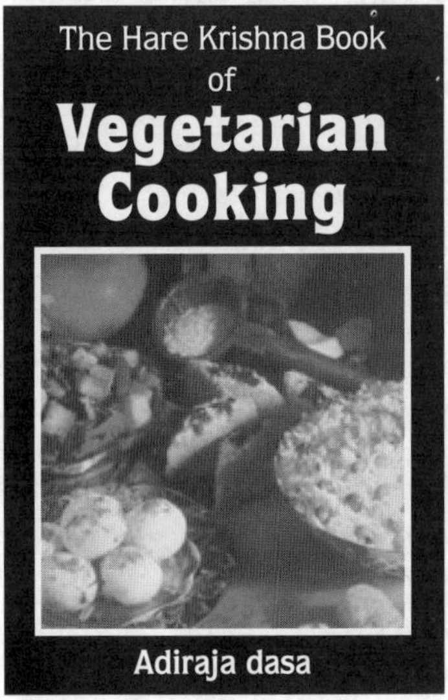

130 kitchen-tested recipes, 300 pages, hardback

US: $11.50 #HKVC

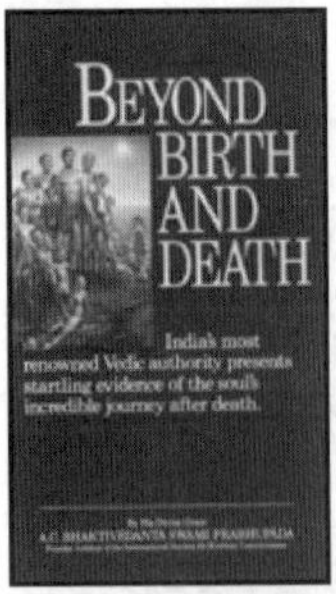

BEYOND BIRTH AND DEATH

What's the self? Can it exist apart from the physical body? If so, what happens to the self at the time of death? What about reincarnation? Liberation? *Beyond Birth and Death* answers these intriguing questions and more.

Softbound, 96 pages

US$1.00 #BBD

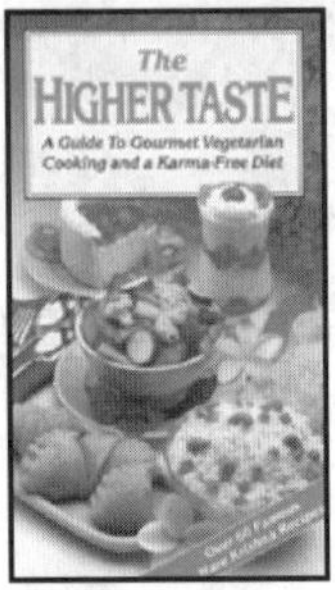

THE HIGHER TASTE

A Guide to Gourmet Vegetarian Cooking and a Karma-Free Diet

Illustrated profusely with black-and-white drawings and eight full-color plates, this popular volume contains over 60 tried and tested international recipes, together with the why's and how's of the Krishna conscious vegetarian life-style.

Softbound, 176 pages

US$1.50 #HT

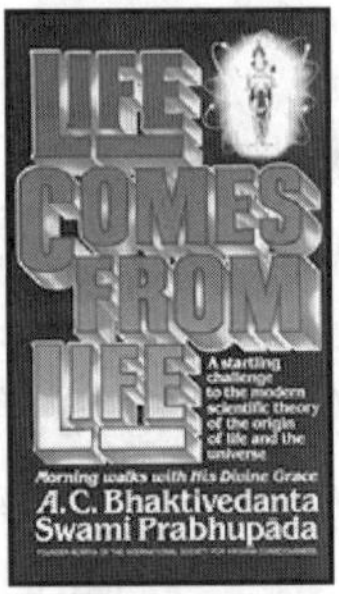

LIFE COMES FROM LIFE

In this historic series of talks with his disciples, Śrīla Prabhupāda uncovers the hidden and blatantly unfounded assumptions that underlie currently fashionable doctrines concerning the origins and purpose of life.

Softbound, 96 pages

US$1.50 #LCFL

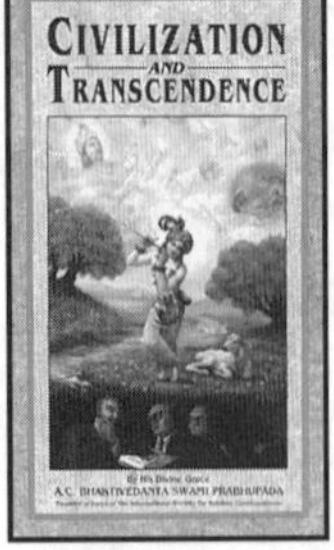

CIVILIZATION AND TRANSCENDENCE

In this book Śrīla Prabhupāda calls the bluff of modern materialistic culture, both East and West. An excerpt: "Modern so-called civilization is simply a dog's race. The dog is running on four legs, and modern people are running on four wheels. The learned, astute person will use this life to gain what he has missed in countless prior lives—namely, realization of self and realization of God."

Softbound, 90 pages

US$1.00 #CT

Posters

Superb Florentino linen embossed prints. All posters are 18 x 24. (Besides the three shown, there are ten others to choose from. Call for our *free* catalog.)

US$3.75 each #POS

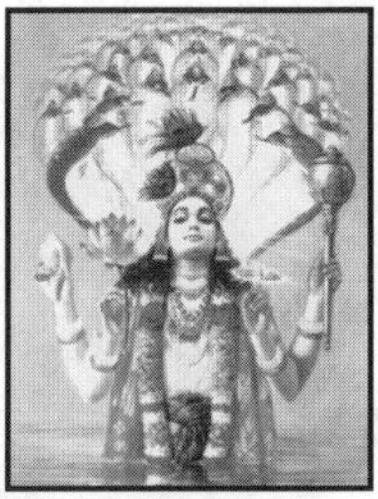

Śrī Viṣṇu

Mantra Meditation Kit

Includes a string of 108 hand-carved *japa* beads, a cotton carrying bag, counter beads, and instructions.

US$5.00
#MMK

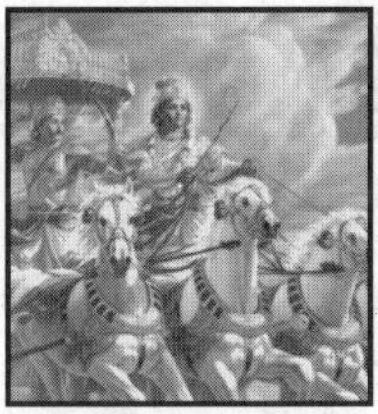

Pārtha Sārathi

The Rādhā-Kṛṣṇa Temple Album

The original Apple LP produced by George Harrison, featuring "Hare Kṛṣṇa Mantra" and the "Govinda" prayers that are played daily in ISKCON temples around the world. On stereo cassette or CD.

US$3.75 for cassette #CC-6
US$11.25 for CD #CD-6

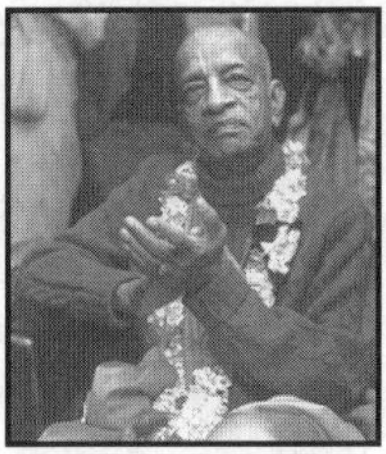

Śrīla Prabhupāda

Śrīla Prabhupāda Chanting Japa

This recording of His Divine Grace A.C. Bhaktivedanta Swami Prabhupāda chanting *japa* is a favorite among young and old devotees alike.

US$2.95 for cassette #JT-1

Incense

Twenty sticks per pack, hand rolled in India. Highest quality, packed in foil.

US$1.50 per pack #INC

ORDER TOLL FREE 1-800-927-4152

Order Form

Make check or money order payable to The Bhaktivedanta Book Trust and send to:

The Bhaktivedanta Book Trust
Dept. POY-H
3764 Watseka Avenue • Los Angeles, CA 90034

Name ______________________________
Please Print
Address ______________________________
City ____________________ ST _____ Zip __________

Code	Description	Qty.	Price	Total

Subtotal US $ __________

CA Sales Tax 8.25% US $ __________

Shipping 15% of Subtotal (minimum $2.00) US $ __________

TOTAL US $ __________

To Place a Credit Card Order Please Call

1-800-927-4152

VISA MasterCard